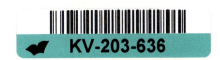

Current Topics in Anaesthesia

General Editors: Stanley A. Feldman
Cyril F. Scurr

2 The Control of Chronic Pain

This book is dedicated to the Pain Relief Foundation

The control of chronic pain

Sampson Lipton, FFA,RCS

Director, The Centre for Pain Relief,
Department of Medical and Surgical Neurology,
Walton Hospital, Liverpool

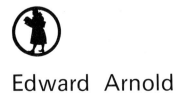

Edward Arnold

© *Sampson Lipton 1979*

First published 1979
by Edward Arnold (Publishers) Ltd
41 Bedford Square, London WC1B 3DQ

British Library Cataloguing in Publication Data
Lipton, Sampson
    The control of chronic pain.—(Current topics in anaesthesia; 2).
    1. Pain
    I. Title II. Series
    616′.047   RB127

ISBN 0-7131-4339-8

Text set in 10/11pt Monophoto Times and
printed in Great Britain by Butler & Tanner Ltd, Frome and London

General preface to series

The current rate of increase of scientific knowledge is such that it is recognized that ... 'ninety per cent of all the existing knowledge which can be drawn upon for the practice of medicine is less than 10 years old'.*

In an acute specialty, such as anaesthesia, failure to keep abreast of advances can seriously effect the standard of patient care. The need for continuing education is widely recognized and indeed it is mandatory in some countries.

However, due to the flood of new knowledge which grows in an exponential fashion greatly multiplying the pool of information every decade, the difficulty that presents itself is that of selecting and retrieving the information that is of immediate value and clinical relevance. This series has been produced in an effort to overcome this dilemma.

By producing a number of authoritative reviews the Current Topics Series has allowed the General Editors to select those in which it is felt there is a particular need for a digest of the large amount of literature, or for a clear statement of the relevance of new information.

By presenting these books in a concise form it should be possible to publish these reviews quickly. Careful selection of authors allows the presentation of mature clinical judgement on the relative importance of this new information.

The information will be clearly presented and, by emphasizing only key references and by avoiding an excess of specialist jargon, the books will, it is hoped, prove to be useful and succinct.

It has been our intention to avoid the difficulties of the large textbooks, with their inevitable prolonged gestation period, and to produce books with a wider appeal than the comprehensive, detailed, and highly specialized monographs. By this means we hope that the Current Topics in Anaesthesia Series will make a valuable contribution by meeting the demands of continuing education in anaesthesia.

S. A. F.
London 1978   C. F. S.

* Education and Training for the Professions.
  Sir Frank Hartley, Wilkinson Lecture,
  Delivered at the Institute of Dental Surgery, 30.1.78
  University of London Bulletin, May 1978, No. 45, p. 3

Preface

This book is written for those doctors, students and other workers already interested in the control and relief of chronic pain, and for those who would like to know more about it. If read quickly from cover to cover, it will give an overall view of current practical methods of pain control and the principles and theories behind this treatment. In a small book such as this, it is not possible to comment on every type of treatment and I mention only those methods which I think are worth further study.

All the techniques mentioned are in use in the British Isles, though not at one clinic. Most of these techniques have been used or are at present in use at the Centre for Pain Relief, Walton Hospital, Liverpool.

There are two areas where pain relief is not satisfactory and I mention them specifically. One is pain in the head and the other is rheumatic pain: it is significant that neither form of pain is associated with lethal diseases. They usually involve either severe pain for short periods with complete recovery in between, or slow steady chronic disability. The first type is treated inadequately because it is intermittent, the second because it is constant. These conditions can often be controlled, or the patients made much more comfortable.

It is amazing to realize that only in recent years has the idea arisen of treating pain as an entity when the underlying medical condition cannot be cured. I believe we are seeing the development of a new specialty, and the question of which specialist should look after problem pain patients is an open question. Anaesthesiologists have pioneered this form of treatment and maybe pain relief will become an acknowledged part of anaesthesia just as intensive therapy now is. All doctors are interested in pain relief but those who mean to treat chronic pain properly must study the basis of treatment and develop the necessary skills, whatever their discipline.

Unfortunately, there is plenty of this work in this field for everyone.
Liverpool, 1979   S. L.

Contents

viii   Contents

Glossary of drugs

Approved names	Proprietary names
Amiphenazole	Daptazole
Amitriptyline	Tryptizol, Saroten, etc. (UK))
	Elavil, Endep, (USA)
*Aspirin (UK)	
Acetylsalicylic acid	
Baclofen	Lioresal
Benorylate	Benoral
Benzocaine	
Bezitramide	Burgodin (Netherlands)
Bupivacaine	Marcain
Carbamazepine	Tegretol
Chlorprocaine	Nesacaine, (USA)
Chlorpromazine	Largactil (UK)
	Chlor PZ, Promachel, Promachlor, etc. (USA)
Clonazepam	Rivotril (UK) Clonopin (USA)
Clonidine	Dixarit (also Catapres)
Cyproheptadine	Periactin
Desmopressin	DDAVP
Dexamethasone	Decadron, Dexa-Cortisyl, Oradexon (UK)
	Dexone, Gammacorten, Deronil, etc. (USA)
Dextromoramide	Palfium
Diazepam	Valium
Diflunisal	Dolobid
Dihydrocodeine	DF 118
Dihydroergotamine	DHE 45, (USA)
Dipipanone	Contained in Diconal
Ergotamine	Femergin (and included in several compound tablets, e.g. Cafergot, Migril).
	Ergomar, (USA)
Ergotamine Inhalation	Medihaler Ergotamine
Etidocaine	Duranest
Fluphenazine	Moditen, Modecate, (UK)
	Permitil, Prolixin, (USA)
Guanethidine	Ismelin
Ibuprofen	Brufen, (UK)
	Motrin, (USA)

* Aspirin is a registered trade mark in some countries.

Approved names	Proprietary names
Idoxuridine	Dendrid, Herpid, Kerecid, Ophthalmidine, (UK)
	Stoxil, (USA)
Indomethacin	Indocid, (UK)
	Indocin, (USA)
Iophendylate	Myodil, (UK)
	Pantopaque, (USA)
Levorphanol	Dromoran, (UK) Levo-Dromoran, (USA)
Lignocaine, (UK)	Xylocaine, Lidothesin, etc. (UK)
Lidocaine, (USA)	Anestacon, Lida-Mantle, etc. (USA)
Methadone	Physeptone, (UK)
	Dolophine, Westadone, (USA)
Methotrimeprazine	Veractil, (UK)
	Levoprome, (USA)
Methylprednisolone Acetate	Depo-Medrone, (UK)
	Depo-Medrol, (USA)
Methysergide	Deseril, (UK)
	Sansert, (USA)
Metrizamide	Amipaque
Morphine	
Nalorphine	Lethidrone, (UK)
	Nalline, (USA)
Naloxone	Narcan
Naproxen	Naprosyn
Neostigmine	Prostigmin
Nitrous Oxide 50% with	Entonox
Oxygen 50%	
Orphenadrine	Disipal, Norflex
Pentazocine	Fortral, (UK) Talwin, (USA)
Pethidine, (UK)	Demerol, (USA)
Meperidine, (USA)	
Phenazocine	Narphen
Phenol	
Phenoperidine	Operidine (N.B. Operidine is a synonym for
	Pethidine in Japan).
Phenylbutazone	Butazolidin, (UK) Azolid, (USA)
Phenytoin	Epanutin, (UK) Dilantin, (USA)
Prednisone	DeCortisyl, Deltacortone, Di-Andreson, (UK)
	Delta-Dome, Lisacort, Orasone, (USA)
Prilocaine	Citanest
Procaine	Novocain, (USA)
Propranolol	Inderal
Reserpine	Serpasil, (UK) Eskaserp, Raurine, Reserpoid,
	etc. (USA)
Sulphinpyrazone, (UK)	Anturan
Sulfinpyrazone, (USA)	
Suxamethonium	Brevidil M, Anectine, (UK) Scoline, Quelicin,
	Sucostrin, (USA)
Tacrine (Tetrahydroaminacrine)	THA
Trichlorofluoromethane 25%	P.R. Spray, Skefron, (UK)
with Dichlorodifluoro-	Similar products in USA include Freon
methane 15%	Genetron and Isotron.

Acknowledgement The glossary was compiled by Mr D. Stobbs, Principal Pharmacist, Walton Hospital, Liverpool. The author wishes to register his thanks to Mr Stobbs.

1

Introduction

An organism becomes aware of its surroundings through their effect on its substance. It is at its own periphery that it is in contact with the environment and it is not surprising that in highly developed organisms certain portions of the peripheral tissues are modified to appreciate changes in these surroundings. Specialized organs develop which appreciate light, sound, pressure and touch; others such as senses of balance and position allow the organism to be aware of itself in relation to the environment. Combined with these is the ability to protect itself against either the environment or a predator. Part of this protection is the appreciation of noxious stimuli.

This appreciation is complicated since a given stimulus, say the application of heat, may at first be pleasant (i.e. the organism is comfortable), then it may become too hot (i.e. uncomfortable but not damaging) and finally the organism may burn and the stimulus is noxious. The alerting system must distinguish between these and also decide what active measure is required to remove the organism from the presence of the noxious stimulus. Is it enough to move the affected part? To move the whole organism? Should it turn and fight, or run away? The prospects for survival have to be assessed very rapidly and action taken.

When noxious stimuli reach consciousness they register as pain. This is not a simple sensation, as it is a combination of many elements including severe discomfort, fear, autonomic changes, reflex movements and attention. The use of the word 'suffering' is often used in relation to persistent severe pain and suggests that there is a mental element attached to it.

A patient who suffers intractable pain from, say, an inoperable cancer has severe, constant and unremitting pain. As mentioned later, this patient will become progressively demoralized, concentrating solely on his pain. If such a patient has a leucotomy and the connections between the frontal regions of the brain and the thalamus are interrupted by surgery, the patient's attitude alters. He will state that the severity and frequency of his pain is unaltered but it no longer worries him. The element of suffering has disappeared.

Normally, the role of pain is beneficial and this is recognized most readily with the occasional child born with a congenital absence of pain. These unfortunates are unable to appreciate the dangers surrounding them and they

1

develop terrible injuries because there is no limiting sensation. They have no fear of fire or heat and will allow themselves to burn or scald without moving away. They will bite the flesh off their fingers and chew their tongues. Without the appreciation of pain they develop fracture after fracture. They are unable to safeguard their bodies since they cannot recognize danger. Even when they are damaged, their relatives and physicians may not recognize the presence of injury for many days owing to the lack of concern shown by the child. Naturally these children die young.

At the other extreme of the pain scale are those patients who, having suffered a minor injury, develop persistent severe burning pain with paroxysmal exacerbations which are unrelieved by normal measures. As time goes by, the adjacent sites may be affected but usually the pain is confined to the original area. Trophic changes in the skin occur with oedema and vasomotor changes. If this occurs in the hand, in a surprisingly short time osteoporosis of the disused bones of fingers and hand appear and the patient adopts a protective position designed to avoid the slightest contact with the affected limb. This particular condition, a reflex sympathetic dystrophy known as Sudeck's atrophy, usually responds to repeated sympathetic block—but not always.

When a noxious stimulus damages peripheral tissues, an electrical discharge occurs and is transmitted through nervous pathways to the spinal cord and thence upwards to the higher brain centres. The situation at which the electrical stimulation is translated into the conscious sensation of pain is unknown but some of the pathways are known and are described shortly. What is important is to realize that the electrical stimulation signifying noxious damage may be suppressed, or enhanced, or have its time relationship changed during transmission. It may persist and spread but, normally, noxious stimulation does none of these things. Thus, any description of pain production and transmission must explain how normal transmission changes to produce abnormal effects.

The explanation begins logically in Chapter 2 with descriptions of simple and excitable cells and then progresses from peripheral to central portions of the c.n.s. Pathological pain is discussed in Chapter 5.

2
Neurophysiology

The cell

All animal tissues consist of closely packed cells and the interstitial fluid which surrounds them. The intracellular fluid and the interstitial fluid are similar in that both contain particles dissolved in water. The boundary between the intracellular and the interstitial fluids, known as the cell membrane, is highly organized and restricts the exchange of substance between the two compartments.

The difference between them is much more striking than the similarities; in particular, there are different concentrations of different ions on the two sides of the membrane and there is an electric potential difference between them. It is thought that ionized substances cross the membrane via water-filled pores, or by carrier molecules limited to the membrane substance.

The intracellular fluid contains K^+ in high concentrations and Cl^- and Na^+ in low concentrations. On the other hand, the interstitial fluid contains high concentrations of Na^+ and Cl^- and low concentrations of K^+ ion. K^+ penetrates the cell membrane fifty times more easily than Na^+, and it is the excess K^+ diffusing out through the cell membrane which produces the trans-membrane voltage by charging the outside of the membrane positively. This positive voltage will then attract Cl^- through the cell wall and this tends to neutralize the membrane charge. The end result is an outward migration of Na^+, Cl^- and H_2O, an increase of K^+, and an electrical gradient which constitutes the membrane potential.

Excitable cells

A normal cell produces a steady transmembrane potential. Some cells—and the neurone is one of them—are unique in being excitable, and a stimulus produces a partial depolarization of the cell membrane by altering the permeability of the membrane to Na^+. An influx of Na^+ then results, and depolarization and a further increased permeability to Na^+ continue in progressive fashion until the membrane is completely depolarized. After an interval, recovery occurs and is known as repolarization.

3

The process produced by a stimulus is known as an impulse; at the same time there is an alteration of voltage which is the action potential. Action potentials spread along the surface membrane of the cell and, if the cell is elongated, spread along the length.

Neurone

A motor neurone has two types of processes: the dendrites and axons. The dendrites are about 1 mm long, are thick at their base, and branch and taper. The axon has a constriction in its initial segment and beyond this increases in diameter, acquires a myelin sheath and in the spinal cord will proceed from the spinal cord into the ventral root. The difference between axons and dendrites is usually apparent as the axon has a uniform diameter, is much longer than the dendrites and seldom gives off collaterals. Thus an action potential, once initiated in a neurone, will spread throughout its surface and progress along the axon.

Synapse

At its termination the axon makes contact with other neurones but is not in direct contact with them as there is a space between, known as a synapse. The terminal branches of pre-synaptic fibres end on both the dendrites and the cell body of the post-synaptic cell, and form small round or oval swellings which are the synaptic knobs or boutons. The cell body has many of these boutons, while on the dendrites their numbers decrease as they divide into terminal branches. The synaptic knob is not part of the cell body. Each has a continuous cell membrane of about 5 nm (50 Å) thick which makes a slight indentation into the cell tissue but between the two membranes there is the synaptic gap which is 20 nm (200 Å) wide. In addition to mitochondria, the knob contains many small rounded structures—the synaptic vesicles   which contain the substances important for synaptic transmission.

Synaptic transmission

Transmission across a synaptic cleft occurs after a sufficiently strong impulse travels along an axon and reaches its termination. At this point an alteration in the concentration of sodium and potassium ions is produced by a change in the permeability of the cell membrane, and the synaptic vesicles within the axon terminal release a chemical transmitter into the synaptic gap which reaches the following neurone. The mechanism has been well studied at the neuromuscular junction where the transmitter substance is acetylcholine. There are many neurotransmitters in the central nervous system, such as glutamic acid, dopamine, norepinephrine, 5-hydroxytryptamine and acetylcholine. There are, without doubt, a number of other transmitter substances and some of these are known to take part in the pain mechanism (Oliveras *et al.*, 1975; Davies and Dray, 1977; Messing and Lytle, 1977).

The various synaptic knobs on, for instance, a single motor neurone do not originate from the same afferent fibre but arise from many different afferent fibres and thus the motor neurone forms the final effector organ upon which many pre-synaptic fibres converge. Activity must occur in many synaptic knobs within a very short time to produce an impulse in the motor neurone. Discharge of the motor neurone results from almost synchronous activity in a number of afferent fibres converging on to that motor neurone. An afferent nerve fibre breaks up into many branches which make synaptic contact with many post-synaptic cells; in this way, although no one single afferent fibre on its own can fire a motor neurone, each afferent fibre takes part in the firing of a series of motor neurones. Thus, on the one hand, there is a convergence of many pre-synaptic fibres on to single cells and, on the other hand, a divergence from one neurone via its many axon fibrils on to a number of cells. It is because of these arrangements that the phenomenon of facilitation occurs.

Facilitation

If two afferent fibres stimulate separately, neither alone will fire a motor neurone, but if both are stimulated together, their effects summate and the neurone may fire. If instead of a single motor neurone (as in this example) a series of motor neurones is visualized, it can be seen how stimulation of one or more afferent fibres in different combinations can produce different effects.

Inhibition

The converse of facilitation is inhibition, where stimulation in the afferent fibre produces change in the post-synaptic neurone, reducing its excitability. In these inhibitory synapses the transmitter substance diffuses across the synaptic cleft, reaches the post-synaptic membrane and makes it less excitable. When a membrane becomes less excitable it is said to be hyperpolarized.

A physical stimulus arriving at an organism's periphery initiates neural action. Stimuli become effective when they are applied to specialized afferent fibre terminals. The physical stimuli include light, mechanical distortion, chemical damage, heat and many others. The specialized afferent fibre terminals are known as receptor structures.

The receptor

This is the peripheral mechanism which transforms a physical stimulus into an electrical change corresponding in its timing and strength to the stimulus producing it. In other words, the receptor acts as a transducer, translating one form of energy into another. Each receptor is specially adapted for detecting particular kinds of energy and thus there are thermoreceptors, chemoreceptors and mechanoreceptors. Some receptors are only responsive to one type of stimulus but, in general terms, most receptors will respond to more than one kind of stimulus, especially when the stimulus intensity increases. Nociceptors respond only to stimuli causing tissue damage, and give rise to pain; most receptors when stimulated by tissue damage also respond with sensation of pain. There is great variability in the anatomical arrangements of receptors seen most clearly in the special sense organs, such as hearing and sight. Nevertheless, some receptors are very simple, consisting of thin unmyelinated prolongations of the original axon, while others form elaborate arrangements with connective tissue capsules or terminate around non-neural cells. Some are specialized to detect a particular stimulus such as mechanical displacement of a hair, but specialization is not invariable; the cornea, for instance, contains only free nerve endings and is sensitive to touch, warmth, cold and pain.

Generator potential

A receptor terminal's response to a simulus is the graded and non-propagated local depolarization known as the generator or receptor potential. A generator potential is directly related to the intensity of the stimulus, and is present only in the terminals; it is usually short-lived. If the stimulus is increased, it will reach threshold level and an action potential will be produced. This is a self-propagating process.

Adaptation

Receptors show adaptation when the stimulus is prolonged, which means that the generator potential decreases during continuous stimulation. Some receptors show only a limited decrease of generator potential during this prolonged stimulation period and are slowly adapting receptors while, in others—the rapidly adapting receptors—adaptation reduces the membrane potential below the firing level. These two types of receptors are also known as tonic and phasic receptors. Phasic receptors signal the beginning and end of a stimulation while tonic receptors signal the presence of a continuous stimulus.

There is no continuous connection between the periphery and the brain; it is important to realize that this is so because it means that conduction through a chain of neurones is not automatic and that the original axon potential message can be modified at each synapse. The pre-synaptic impulse travelling along the axon initiates a new impulse in the post-synaptic cell. Action potentials in a chain of neurones are conducted in one direction, and neural activity can be amplified or suppressed at the synapse. A repetitive discharge in a following neurone occurs after a synchronous volley is delivered over the pre-synaptic pathway. However, there is a refractory period between each stimulus producing an action potential; while the refractoriness is present, there is a limit on the accurate transmission of a signal so therefore the post-synaptic neurone may not accurately respond to each of a series of repetitive pre-synaptic discharges. In general terms, the longer the chain of neurones and the greater the number of synapses, the less chance is there of the end frequency corresponding accurately to the initiating frequency. That patterns of discharge are altered passing across the various synapses in a chain of neurones is most significant in understanding how abnormal patterns can develop under some circumstances and may then be interpreted as pain.

The spinal cord

Sensations generated in the periphery are carried to the central nervous system (c.n.s.) in two ways: by the dorsal columns and by the anterolateral tracts. The dorsal column consists of large myelinated primary afferent fibres (group II) which originate in low threshold, tactile and articular mechanoreceptors; at their point of entry into the spinal cord the cutaneous mechanoreceptors give off collaterals to the dorsal horn. Unmyelinated peripheral afferent fibres (group IV or C) terminate in the substantia gelatinosa of the dorsal horn, and small myelinated afferents (group III) terminate in the nucleus proprius. The nucleus proprius is lamina V of Rexed (1954) and spinothalamic fibres arise in this layer.

Laminae

Rexed showed that the cells of the grey matter in the spinal cord are arranged in nine laminae, labelled I–IX, from dorsal to ventral spinal cord (Fig. 2.1). A tenth lamina surrounds the central canal. Lamina I corresponds to the marginal zone, and laminae II and III to the substantia gelatinosa. These form one section in the spinal cord and some group III and IV fibres terminate in this region. It is believed that group III and IV fibres, entering the marginal zone and substantia gelatinosa, are those carrying pain impulses. Laminae IV, V and VI are known as the nucleus proprius, and the small myelinated fibres (group III) which are activated by pinprick and hot and cold receptors terminate there. Laminae VII and VIII correspond to the nucleus intermedius and give rise to the spinoreticular fibres. Finally, there is lamina IX which is the ventral horn and the output of these nerve cells form the ventral root.

Each lamina is connected to the succeeding lamina, and stimulation from the cells in each lamina converges on the next lamina. Thus, if there is sufficient stimulation in the group III fibres entering the nucleus proprius, lamina V cells will be activated to produce stimulation travelling over the spinothalamic fibres. The stimulation in this section of the laminae is not usually sufficient to stimulate successive laminae into activity but if, for instance, group III and IV fibres entering the marginal zone and substantia gelatinosa carry a high level of activity through noxious stimulation of the skin, while other group III fibres entering the nucleus proprius also carry a high level of stimulation because of peripheral activity, then the combined stimulation from I, II and III, and IV, V and VI laminae may be sufficient to stimulate VII and VIII in the nucleus intermedius and fire cells connected with the spinoreticular fibres. In this way a much greater stimulatory output is produced. In other words, the organization of the spinal laminae is such as to ensure the upward transmission of information if that stimulation increases above a normal level.

Transmission of stimulation—that is, of information—in the spinal cord is not simply a one-for-one arrangement. There is a differential transmission which makes use of convergence and divergence in the synaptic connections between nerve cells and this arrangement ensures that minor unimportant

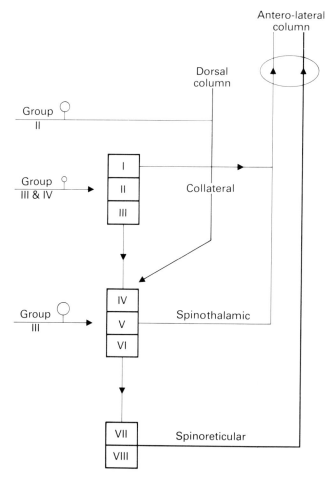

Fig. 2.1   Rexed laminae. I, marginal zone; II and III, substantia gelatinosa; IV, V and VI, nucleus proprius; VII and VIII, nucleus intermedius.

stimulation can be suppressed while other high level activity is summated (Bowsher, 1977).

Gate control (Fig. 2.2)

Mention has already been made of collaterals of dorsal column fibres, and it is believed that these collaterals are segmental and synapse in lamina IV. In a way which is not yet completely understood, they exert an inhibitory effect on the transmission of nerve impulses from the substantia gelatinosa across lamina IV to successive layers of the spinal cord. It is probable that this mechanism constitutes the basis of the gate control system described by Melzack and Wall in 1965 (Kerr 1976), which is discussed below.

According to this theory, peripheral damage activates not only nerve fibres which stimulate the substantia gelatinosa and nucleus proprius but also large myelinated axons in the dorsal column fibres. Collaterals from these carry inhibitory stimulation which tends to block some of the stimulation travelling from the substantia gelatinosa to the nucleus proprius. In this way painful sensation can be reduced.

In Chapter 11 it will be shown that inhibiting stimulation along the collaterals of the dorsal column fibres can be augmented to reduce chronic pain. Also it can now be seen that a reduction in large myelinating fibres or hyperactivity along unmyelinated C fibres will perpetuate painful conditions.

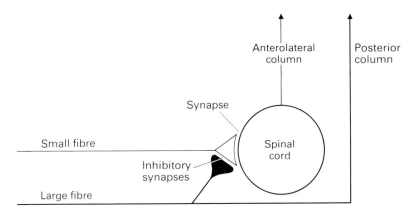

Fig. 2.2 Gate control (diagrammatic).

Just as there is summation of stimulation through mechanisms such as the spinal laminae, so is there summation and inhibition of onward transmission in the brain stem and higher centres. Reticular fibres and neurones form a lattice in the brain stem, and the ascending and descending neurones and fibres are intermingled with interconnections between them. The reticular fibres collateralize widely and one neurone will have a wide field of secondary neurones to each of which it will give a small number of connections.

Sensory pathway

Afferent impulses reach the spinal cord in the posterior horns and axons carrying sensations of pain, heat and cold, cross the cord to the anterolateral quadrant and then ascend, forming the spinothalamic tract. These fibres reach the posterolateral ventral nucleus of the thalamus. There are other nerve fibres in the anterolateral white column and these form a multisynaptic spinothalamic pathway connecting the spinal cord with reticular nuclei in the medulla, midbrain, tectum and thalamus. This second pathway with its diffuse connections with the reticular system probably serves as an alerting system and is a phylogenetically older system than the first.

In addition, there is another pathway formed by large myelinated fibres in the posterior nerve root which run in the posterior columns of the spinal cord and synapse in the gracile and cuneate nuclei of the medulla. They then cross the midline and reach the posterolateral nucleus of the thalamus through the medial lemniscus. This pathway was originally believed to be concerned with fine discrimination such as joint sense, vibration sense and two-point discrimination. Wall (1970) suggested this third pathway is connected with those discriminative sensations which need to be interpreted after a motor movement. This distinguishes their function from the other pathways carrying sensations which are received in passive fashion.

Thalamus

Pain reaches consciousness at the level of the thalamus. This is not one nucleus but a series of nuclei, and a number of these are known to be involved in pain appreciation. Ascending reticular fibres form two groups, one of which is mainly distributed to the intralaminar nuclei of the thalamus, the other passing to the hypothalamus. The spinothalamic tracts terminate in the posterolateral ventral nuclei of the thalamus before relaying onwards, and the posterior column fibres also terminate in the thalamus. Thus it can be seen that all sensory fibres converge on the thalamus.

Descending control

Not only is there ascending transmission from the periphery to those levels of the higher centres where the stimulation reaches consciousness but there is also a descending control over sensory input. There are direct and indirect pathways exerting a modulating influence which exist at every level of the brain stem and spinal cord, and include the dorsal horn of the spinal cord where they form part of the gate control mechanism.

Pain can be suppressed under conditions of stress. This phenomenon is well documented. It can also be suppressed under many other conditions which include hypnosis, alpha conditioning, religious ecstasy and electrical stimulation.

References

Bowsher, D. (1977). The anatomo-physiology of pain. In: *Persistent Pain*, vol. 1, p. 1. Ed. by S. Lipton. Academic Press, London and New York.
Davies, J. and Dray, A. (1977). Substance P and opiate receptors. *Nature* **268**, 351–352.
Kerr, F. W. L. (1976). Segmental circuitry and spinal cord nociceptive mechanisms. In: *Advances in Pain Research and Therapy*, vol. 1, pp. 75–89. Ed. by J. J. Bonica and D. Albe-Fessard. Raven Press, New York.
Melzack, R. and Wall, P. D. (1965). Pain mechanisms: a new theory. *Science* **150**, 971–979.

Messing, B. B. and Lytle, L. D. (1977). Serotonin-containing neurons: their possible role in pain and analgesia. *Pain* **4**, 1–22.

Oliveras, J. L., Redjemi, F., Guilbaud, G. and Besson, J. M. (1975). Analgesia induced by electrical stimulation of the inferior centralis nucleus of the raphe in the cat. *Pain* **1**, 139–145.

Rexed, B. (1954). The cytoarchitectonic organization of the spinal cord in the cat. *Journal of Comparative Neurology* **23**, 259.

Wall, P. D. (1970). The sensory and motor role of impulses travelling in the dorsal columns towards cerebral cortex. *Brain* **93**, 505–524.

3

The gate control theory of pain

Stimulation of peripheral receptors in the skin is normally interpreted at the higher centres as pinprick, touch or hot and cold sensations. If the stimulation is so intense that tissue damage occurs, then these sensations are interpreted as pain. It must be appreciated that the electrical stimulation travelling along peripheral nerves from stimulated peripheral receptors is not pain. What is being transmitted from receptor to peripheral nerve, to spinal cord, to brain stem and on up to those centres in the cerebrum which interpret the sensation, is information. If this information is of a particular variety it will be interpreted as pain. Sensation from the periphery is transmitted in a code which is translated by the central nervous system in such a way as to give the position of the stimulus in relation to the body, and also the type and intensity of the stimulus. If this is a noxious stimulus then that also is included in the information. Unfortunately, no single code is used throughout the central nervous system and it has to be realized that at each synapse the code is modulated. It is possible that chronic pain is appreciated because of damage to a section of this system and either a particular stimulus is coded incorrectly or the code is translated incorrectly.

In the past there have been a number of theories of pain and these can briefly be divided into two types: those, known as specificity theory, which postulated a pain pathway on a purely anatomical basis; and the pattern theory, in which the basic idea was that pain occurred as a result of patterns of stimulation which were interpreted at higher discriminating centres. Neither of these two theories is correct; the specific theory cannot explain, for instance, perseverating pain or the long delays before the appreciation of some pains or their referral over wide areas. The pattern theory is obviously incorrect because there are definite known anatomical pain pathways. The third theory is the gate control theory (Melzack and Wall, 1965) which suggests how transmission from the periphery to the central nervous system is modified. The theory attempts to explain how an identical stimulation does not even reach consciousness on one occasion, on another will be interpreted as pinprick and on another as pain. There was considerable previous work before Melzack and Wall put forward their theory. Much of the earlier work was designed to explain two phenomena: the dorsal root reflex and the dorsal root potential. The dorsal root reflex orginates in the posterior horn cells and consists of a nervous discharge which is conducted antidromically in peripheral nerves. Wall (1959) showed that depolarization of afferent fibre terminals, if great enough, would produce spontaneous impulses which would travel along a nerve fibre. The dorsal root reflex is due to such impulses running peripherally in the posterior nerve roots.

In 1938 (Barron and Matthews) showed that the dorsal root potential is a depolarization of afferent fibre terminals in the grey matter. Transmission cannot take place orthodromically when these are depolarized and thus the afferent nerve is partially or intermittently blocked. This effect is still present when the particular nerve root is sectioned because nerve input into adjacent nerve fibres will continue the activity. In 1964 Wall believed that an afferent fibre terminal could be held in a partially depolarized state and then it could act as a trigger mechanism on which other incoming impulses acted. Eccles called this phenomenon pre-synaptic inhibition.

The gate control theory of Melzack and Wall is the basis of modern pain theory. It provides the best explanation so far, as to why pain behaves in the way it does. In this theory it is postulated that large diameter A fibres (A-β fibres), the smaller diameter A fibres (A-δ fibres) and the C fibres are all activated during any noxious stimulation of peripheral receptors. The theory suggests that, at the spinal cord level, there is a 'gate'. This gate under certain circumstances allows pain stimulation to pass through it and impinge on the higher centres. It is believed that small nerve fibre stimulation tends to open the gate and that stimulation along larger fibres tends to close it. What is meant by this is not that the gate closes tight, or opens wide, but that activity along these two types of fibres depresses or facilitates synaptic transmission of pain sensation at spinal cord level. The gate control theory also postulated that this type of gate would exist at all levels of the spinal cord and not only on the pre-synaptic side. Melzack and Wall expected to find similar gates at post-synaptic level and at other levels in the central nervous system. Not only was the gate under local control from the periphery but there was also modulation of the gate through a central descending control mechanism. Thus, cortical and subcortical supraspinal neurones could modulate the gate and this modulation occurred very rapidly. It was thought that one possible mechanism for this rapid ascending and descending pathway could be through the large, rapidly conducting fibres of the dorsal column.

Discussion of the gate control theory

The work leading to the gate control theory was based on the use of electrical stimulation methods in sensory physiology; this work was carried out on small mammals. It does not necessarily follow that what occurs in these experimental animals also occurs in man. For instance, the cat is used in many neurophysiological stimulation studies, and the spinocervical tract which is well developed in this animal has been suggested as a supplementary or possibly main pathway for pain sensation. In the monkey its size is reduced while in man only an occasional neurone related to this system can be found.

When physiologists refer to the threshold of nerve fibres they mean threshold to electrical stimulation under their experimental conditions, and these are not physiological stimuli. Physiological stimuli are initiated at peripheral receptors, and each modality of sensation travels over one size of nerve fibre. Electrical stimulation is made at the middle of a nerve and it travels in both directions, unlike a physiological stimulation. It will also stimulate all the nerve fibres present, which causes the large myelinated nerve fibres to fire first and the non-myelinated fibres last. They will always fire in the same order because they are initiated by a volley of impulses. This is unlike normal stimuli, which tend to have a gradual onset, wax and wane gradually, and travel over a number of nerve roots and not one alone.

The reason for the use of electrical methods is fairly obvious as it is reproducible and averaging techniques allow background noise to be eliminated. It also allows waves of stimuli to be identified and timed. There are a number of compartments to the gate control theory and peripheral stimulation passes through these before pain stimulation is transmitted onwards. Initially there must be ongoing activity, due to proprioceptive and cutaneous stimuli, which itself produces further activity. Then there is the relative balance between the activity of large and small nerve fibres. Next is the intrinsic neurone which forms the link between the periphery and the brain and is called the T cell or transmission cell. The substantia gelatinosa controls the membrane potential of the peripheral afferent fibres by pre-synaptic inhibition, with large and small fibre afferent input acting in different directions. Input from large fibres produces pre-synaptic inhibition of the peripheral input while input from small fibres reduces or prevents this pre-synaptic inhibition.

There were additional features to the theory in that it proposed that there were descending fibres from the brain which could produce pre-synaptic inhibition at segmental level and that this could occur through large afferent fibres in the posterior columns (or spinocervical tracts). In normal circumstances pain does not occur because large fibre activity is present, causing pre-synaptic inhibition and preventing summation with small fibre activity. Thus, there is no onward transmission to the T cell.

Certain parts of the gate control theory are accepted, certain parts are as yet unproven, and certain parts are not accepted. Before going on to expand a little on this, it must be stated that a theory is important because, to paraphrase Nathan (1976), 'the ideas behind it need to be fruitful, they do not have to be right'. The gate control theory explained and emphasized that pain does not always occur following peripheral stimulation and can occur as a result of the stimulation of fibres unrelated to the painful process. It is now known that the actual physiological and anatomical facts relating to the gate control theory are more complicated than was originally considered and vary in some ways from the original concept. This does not invalidate the theory but merely extends it.

The T cell is a conjectural structure in the gate theory but it is likely that it does exist in lamina V, this being the lamina from which the spinothalamic fibres arise (Dilly, Wall and Webster, 1968; Pomeranz, Wall and Weber,

1968; Hillman and Wall, 1969). They can arise in other laminae but the major concentration is in lamina V (Trevino, Coulter and Willis, 1973; Price and Mayer, 1975).

The posterior root terminals are subjected to pre-synaptic inhibition by the terminals of afferent fibres on the posterior column nuclei (Andersen, Eccles and Schmidt, 1962; Andersen et al., 1964; Schmidt, 1965; Andersen, Etholm and Gordon, 1968; Jabbur and Banna, 1968, 1970). This appears to be physiological fact but the histological system in which this would be produced has not yet been elucidated, though recently Kerr (1976) has suggested neuronal circuits by which primary afferents exert effects on gelatinosal cells which could then produce inhibition of a marked degree. Iggo (1976) points out that it was not possible to say whether the mechanisms of the inhibitory action in the dorsal horn he studied are pre-synaptic, post-synaptic or both. He comments that there are at least two mechanisms involved in afferent synaptic inhibition. One acts through a glycine transmitter site; the other, which has a longer latency, acts through a γ-aminobutyric transmitter site.

It is crucial to the gate theory that there is a positive phase in the dorsal root potential; in other words, that hyperpolarization exists. This is not accepted by some investigators. For instance, depolarization and hyperpolarization were found by Sessle and Dubner (1971) in cat afferent trigeminal nerve fibres; Gregor and Zimmermann (1972) found that afferent C fibres produced pre-synaptic depolarization in myelinated fibres and not hyperpolarization; and Zimmermann (1968), Franz and Iggo (1968), and Schmidt (1972) failed to find any hyperpolarization of the afferent terminals.

Another important assertion in the gate theory is that the opposing effects result from small and large fibre afferent input. Recent work does not support this concept (Vyklický et al., 1969; Mendell, 1972, 1973; Rudomin et al., 1974; Nathan and Rudge, 1974) in the fashion described in the gate control theory but there is no doubt that large afferent fibres do produce inhibition on slowly conducting fibres at some places in the central nervous system (Noordenbos, 1959).

From the gate control theory it must be axiomatic that any pathological condition in which the numbers of large afferent fibres are reduced in relation to small ones must produce pain. If it does not, then there is a large gap in the basis of the theory. Thus, post-herpetic neuralgia is explained on the basis of a a relative reduction in large fibres (Noordenbos, 1959; Lourie and King, 1966). However, in other conditions such as polyneuropathy there is a relative increase in the small fibres without pain being produced, while in thallium neuropathy it is the small fibres which are reduced, with a relative increase of large fibres, yet this is a very painful condition (Nathan, 1976).

There is selective inhibition of supraspinal origin which can shut down transmission from nociceptors while leaving mechanoreceptor conduction almost unimpaired and there may be a number of sources of this inhibition, such as the cerebral cortex or the median raphe nuclei (Iggo, 1976) (see Chapter 4). The descending axons are dopaminergic and if they are depleted of 5-HT there is a reduction in the analgesic effect of morphine. This suggests that the gate control theory is only part of the pain control and transmission system and that, rather than look at the gate theory as an entity in itself, it should be regarded as the initial portion of a total theory which will be extended and evaluated in due course over many years.

References

Andersen, P., Eccles, J. C. and Schmidt, R. F. (1962). Presynaptic inhibition in the cuneate nucleus. *Nature* **194**, 741–743.

Andersen, P., Eccles, J. C., Schmidt, R. F. and Yokota, T. (1964). Slow potential waves produced in the cuneate nucleus by cutaneous volleys and by cortical stimulation. *Journal of Neurophysiology* **27**, 78–91.

Andersen, P., Etholm, B. and Gordon, G. (1968). Presynaptic depolarisation of dorsal column fibres by adequate stimulation. *Journal of Physiology* **194**, 83–84.

Barron, D. H. and Matthews, B. H. C. (1938). The interpretation of potential changes in the spinal cord. *Journal of Physiology* **92**, 276–321.

Dilly, P. N., Wall, P. D. and Webster, K. E. (1968). Cells of origin of the spino-thalamic tract in cat and rat. *Experimental Neurology* **21**, 550–562.

Eccles, J. C., Schmidt, R. F. and Willis, W. D. (1963). Depolarisation of the central terminals of cutaneous afferent fibres. *Journal of Neurophysiology* **26**, 646–661.

Franz, D. N. and Iggo, A. (1968). Dorsal root potentials and ventral root reflexes evoked by non myelinated fibres. *Science, New York* **162**, 1140–1142.

Gregor, M. and Zimmermann, M. (1972). Characteristics of spinal neurones responding to cutaneous myelinated and unmyelinated fibres. *Journal of Physiology* **221**, 556–576.

Hillman, P. and Wall, P. D. (1969). Inhibitory and excitatory factors influencing the receptive fields of lamina 5 spinal cord cells. *Experimental Brain Research* **9**, 284–306.

Iggo, A. (1976). Peripheral and spinal 'pain' mechanisms and their modulation. In: *Advances in Pain Research and Therapy*, Vol. 1, p. 381. Ed. by J. J. Bonica and D. Albe-Fessard. Raven Press, New York.

Jabbur, S. J. and Banna, N. R. (1968). Presynaptic inhibition of cuneate transmissions by widespread cutaneous inputs. *Brain Research* **10**, 273–276.

Jabbur, S. J. and Banna, N. R. (1970). Widespread cutaneous inhibition in dorsal column nuclei. *Journal of Neurophysiology* **33**, 616–624.

Kerr, F. W. L. (1976). Segmental circuitry and spinal cord nociceptive mechanisms. In: *Advances in Pain Research and Therapy*, Vol. 1, p. 75. Ed. by J. J. Bonica and D. Albe-Fessard. Raven Press, New York.

Lourie, H. and King, R. B. (1966). Sensory and neurohistological correlates of cutaneous hyperpathia. *Archives of Neurology, Chicago* **14**, 313–320.

Melzack, R. and Wall, P. D. (1965). Pain mechanisms: a new theory. *Science* **150**, 971–979.

Mendell, L. (1972). Properties and distribution of peripherally evoked pre-synaptic hyperpolarisation in cat lumbar spinal cord. *Journal of Physiology* **226**, 769–792.

Mendell, L. (1973). Two negative dorsal root potentials evoke a positive dorsal root potential. *Brain Research* **55**, 199–202.

Nathan, P. W. (1976). Critical review of gate control theory. *Brain* **99**, 123–158.

Nathan, P. W. and Rudge, P. (1974). Testing the gate-control theory of pain in man. *Journal of Neurology, Neurosurgery and Psychiatry* **37**, 1366–1372.

Noordenbos, W. (1959). *Pain*, pp. 34–42. Elsevier, Amsterdam.

Pomeranz, B., Wall, P. D. and Weber, W. V. (1969). Cord cells responding to fine myelinated afferent from viscera, muscle and skin. *Journal of Physiology* **199**, 511–532.

Price, D. D. and Mayer, D. S. (1975). Neurophysiological characterization of the anterolateral quadrant neurons subserving pain in *M. mulatta*. *Pain* **1**, 59–72.

Rudomin, P., Nunez, R., Madrid, J. and Burke, R. E. (1974). Primary afferent hyperpolarization and presynaptic facilitation of Ia afferent terminals induced by large cutaneous fibres. *Journal of Neurophysiology* **37**, 413–429.

Schmidt, R. F. (1965). Präsynaptische Hemmung im Nucleus cuneatus der Katze. *Pflügers Archiv für die gesamte Physiologie des Menschen und der Tiere* **278**, 78–79.

Schmidt, R. F. (1972). The gate control theory of pain; an unlikely hypothesis. In: *Pain*, pp. 124–7. Ed. by R. Janzen, W. D. K. Ridel, A. Hertz and C. Steichele. Churchill Livingstone, London.

Sessle, B. J. and Dubner, R. (1971). Presynaptic depolarization and hyperpolarization of trigeminal primary and thalamic afferents. In: *Oral–Facial Sensory and Motor Mechanisms*. Ed. by R. Dubner and Y. Kawamura. Appleton-Century-Crofts, New York.

Trevino, D. L., Coulter, J. D. and Willis, W. D. (1973). Location of cells of origin of spinothalamic tract in lumbar enlargement of monkey. *Journal of Neurophysiology* **36**, 750–761.

Vyklický, L., Rudomin, P., Zajac, F. E. and Burke, R. E. (1969). Primary afferent depolarization evoked by a painful stimulus. *Science* **165**, 184–186.

Wall, P. D. (1959). Repetitive discharge of neurons. *Journal of Neurophysiology* **22**, 305–320.

Wall, P. D. (1964). Presynaptic control of impulses at the first central synapse in the cutaneous pathway. *Progress in Brain Research* **12**, 92–115.

Zimmermann, M. (1968). Dorsal root potentials after C fiber stimulation. *Science, New York* **160**, 896–898.

4

The endogenous opiates

The use of opium as an analgesic substance in the relif of pain has been known for 2000 years. In fact, the word opium comes from the Greek word 'opion' which means poppy juice. Crude opium preparations had long enjoyed widespread use, but by the 1850s pure morphine, an alkaloid isolated from opium, was being used.

However, morphine and other opiates used for analgesia produced opiate addiction and this became a significant social problem. Much effort and large amounts of money have been spent by pharmacologists to develop an opium-like substance which does not have addictive properties. Many opiate drugs have been produced which in their time were believed to be non-addictive, but gradually it became obvious that such drugs were, in fact, addictive.

There are a number of facts which suggest that all opiates have features in common and that they have their effect at specific sites. First, most opiates have two or more chemical forms, the two basic forms existing as optical isomers. Thus opiates have a mirror image molecule which is identical in chemical composition and these optical isomers are distinguished by the direction in which they rotate the plane of polarized light. Most active substances in the human body are laevorotatory, that is they rotate the plane of polarized light to the left. Opiate substances are similar and it is usually only the laevorotatory isomers of opiates which relieve pain and produce addiction. In other words, the opiate molecule is stereo-specific, and this supports the idea of one specific binding site on to which the opiate receptor can fit. The mirror image dextrorotatory isomer does not fit and has no effect.

Another feature suggesting a specific site of action is that the opiate substances produce their effects at low concentrations.

Further, it would be reasonable to expect that opiate substances, if they act at a single receptor site, would have similar chemical formulae and such proves to be the case. Morphine and other opiates have a rigid T-shaped structure which, amongst other features, contains a hydroxyl group and a nitrogen atom.

In addition, the opiate substances or agonists can be modified to form antagonists or substances which block the analgesic and other effects of the agonists without producing any analgesic and similar effects themselves. A com-

18

mon example of an alteration of this type is the substitution of an allyl group for the methyl group in morphine. This converts morphine into nalorphine, which is an antagonist to morphine (Fig. 4.1). Nalorphine in small doses also has a very rapid action and it is likely that the antagonist occupies the same opiate receptor site as morphine and thus blocks the action of morphine.

By using radioactive methods, high affinity binding sites for opiates were found in rat brain and guinea-pig intestine. The radioactive material used was labelled naloxone (Pert and Snyder, 1973). The fact that there are receptor sites in guinea-pig intestine fitted in well with the known effects on the intestine of opiates and also provided a useful laboratory indicator. The indicator used was the ability of different opiates to inhibit the contraction of guinea-pig intestine. This ability was compared with the ability of naloxone

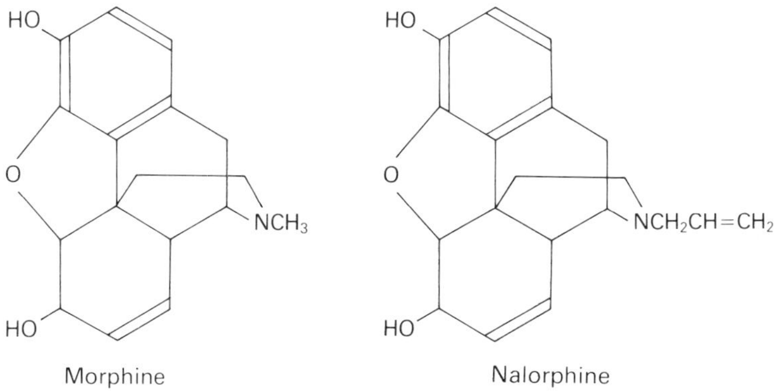

Morphine   Nalorphine

Fig. 4.1   Agonist and antagonist.

to inhibit binding to the guinea-pig intestine. The relative agonist–antagonist binding power to the receptor varies with the concentration of the sodium ion.

Snyder and his co-workers developed a 'sodium index'. This represents the ratio of the concentration of the particular drug required to prevent the binding of naloxone to the opiate receptor by 50 per cent in the presence of sodium, compared to that concentration of the drug required to have the same effect in the absence of sodium. It seems that the sodium index gives an accurate prediction as to whether the drug is an opiate agonist or antagonist. Opiate antagonists such as naloxone have a sodium index of 1 or less and are pure antagonists. Nalorphine, which has both agonist and antagonist properties, has a sodium index of 2·5; pentazocine, which is the only narcotic substance recognized by the World Health Organization as being non-addictive, has a sodium index between 3 and 7. Those drugs which have only a narcotic effect—i.e. those which are pure opiate agonists—have sodium indexes of between 12 and 60. This index and the effect on contraction of the guinea-pig intestine allow a screening process for new agonist–antagonist substances.

The opiate receptor sites outlined by the technique of binding a radioactively labelled agonist to a receptor site and then using autoradiography of brain sections (Pert and Snyder, 1973; Simon, Hiller and Edelman, 1973; Terenius, 1973; Simantov, Showman and Snyder, 1976; Atweh and Kuhar, 1977) showed that the receptor sites are positioned near synapses. In the spinal cord they are found in the marginal zone and substantia gelatinosa of the dorsal horn, and in the descending spinal trigeminal nucleus. At higher levels they occur in the parabrachial nuclei, the ventral median raphe, the superior colliculus and the pretectal nuclei. All these form part of the palaeospinothalamic pain pathway. These receptor sites to opiates have been demonstrated to be present in vetebrates but absent in invertebrates (Snyder, 1977).

Opiate receptor binding was also found in the amygdala, the corpus striatum and the hypothalamus which form part of the limbic system and relate to emotions. It is possible that activity of these areas accounts for the euphoric and addictive effects of opiates. Similar binding sites are also found in the gut.

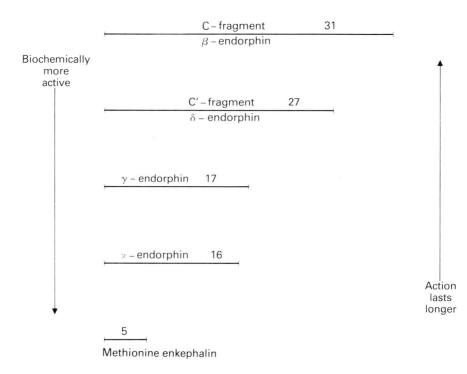

Fig. 4.2   Endogenous opiates, indicating the number of amino-acids in each substance.

The endogenous opiate (Fig 4.2)

From the evidence mentioned above it was obvious to the physiologists and others working in this field that an endogenous opiate must exist, and Hughes *et al.* (1975) found two related pentapeptides—methionine enkephalin and leucine enkephalin—with activity at these sites. These substances have chains short enough to synthesize, and it was shown that they have the same opiate activity and side effects as morphine.

They have a very short duration of action, being broken down very rapidly, while their opiate action is antagonized by naloxone. By immunofluorescent technique, Elde *et al.* (1976) showed that enkephalinergic axons existed in the c.n.s. at the opiate binding sites mentioned previously and they were also found in plexuses in the gut. It would appear that from this and other evidence that the enkephalins are neurotransmitter substances. The axons associated with these substances are very short except in the striatum.

Methionine enkephalin is formed by the breakdown of pituitary β-lipotropin together with another substance known as the C-fragment (now called β-endorphin) which is a much larger fragment of β-lipotropin.

A series of related substances have now been isolated which have opiate agonist activity. The endorphins have longer chains than the enkephalins with β-endorphin consisting of 31 amino-acids. It is present in the hypothalamus, the thalamus and other areas but not in the spinal cord. Enkephalin is rapidly destroyed; in fact, it is destroyed as rapidly as acetylcholine, and because of this is ineffective when injected into the ventricles of the brain. Endorphin, on the contrary, is not so rapidly destroyed and is potent when injected into the ventricles.

Substance P

This substance, now believed to be a neurotransmitter, was discovered by von Euler and Gaddum in 1931. It was isolated from gut in the course of their work on peptides, and is called substance P merely for convenience as it is a powder and the 'P' refers to this property and has no other significance. Vale *et al.* (1975) isolated another peptide, somatostatin, from brain. Of the two, substance P is by far the more common and Hökfelt *et al* (1976) found that 20 per cent of cells in the trigeminal and spinal dorsal root ganglia in the rat were substance P related. The cell bodies of these neurones were small and associated with unmyelinated peripheral fibres. Somatostatin was found in other cells in the dorsal root ganglia but nothing further is known about somatostatin at the present time. However, much further important information for pain transmission is known about substance P positive neurones (SP positive). Their central processes are distributed to laminae I and II of the spinal cord and the descending trigeminal nucleus, and scarcely any are found in the ventral horn.

Substance P is a neurotransmitter substance, and Jessell and Iversen (1977) showed that substance P is released by a calcium-dependent depolarization by potassium ions. In addition, there is evidence (Henry, 1975, 1976) that when noxious peripheral stimuli activate dorsal horn neurones, substance P is produced. Thus substance P appears to be the neurotransmitter substance released by small primary peripheral afferents which transmit painful stimuli.

Jessell and Iversen (1977) found that in the rat, transmission from substance P containing primary afferents is blocked by morphine or enkephalin and pretreatment with naloxone will prevent this.

Enkephalin and substance P (Fig 4.3)

It now seems possible to combine the information available. At spinal cord level noxious stimuli entering the spinal cord stimulate dorsal horn neurones by releasing substance P and normally transmission then progresses to lamina V and up the spinal cord. However, there are inhibitory enkephalinergic interneurones in the substantia gelatinosa which act on the terminals of the unmyelinated primary afferents. These produce enkephalin at their terminals

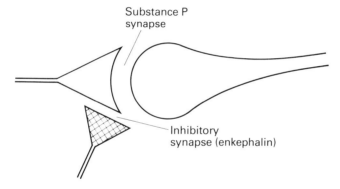

Fig. 4.3   Mode of action of substance P and enkephalin.

and this blocks the production of substance P, thus inhibiting pain transmission. There may well be a chain of neurones forming the inhibitory pathway and it is most likely that the inhibitory enkephalinergic interneurone might be activated by the segmental collaterals of large, low-threshold myelinated primary afferents which form the dorsal columns. This would explain why transcutaneous and dorsal column stimulation (DCS) neuromodulation are effective.

Descending control

So far, the information available offers an explanation of pain transmission mechanisms at spinal cord levels, with particular reference to laminae I and II. However, it is known that stimulation of certain areas of the brain—

especially the periaqueductal grey matter (PAG)—produces analgesia (Mayer *et al.*, 1971), and morphine in miniscule quantities in this region is a most effective method of producing analgesia (Pert and Yaksh, 1974). Cells in the PAG of the rat contain enkephalin (Hökfelt *et al.*, 1977), and morphine and methionine enkephalin produce increased activity of PAG neurones while analgesia is present. Electrodes have been implanted in this region (Richardson and Akil, 1977; Hosobuchi, Adams and Linchitz, 1977) and the analgesic effect produced by stimulation of these electrodes can be reversed by naloxone.

There is a projection from the midline raphe nuclei to the spinal cord and the trigeminal spinal nucleus which appears to be the effective final common pathway for the suppression of pain. The raphe neurones have unmyelinated axons and are serotoninergic with 5-hydroxytryptamine (5-HT) as the transmitter. Blocking these nerve fibres by destruction of the raphe nuclei removes the effect of systemic morphine (Proudfitt and Anderson, 1975). There are enkephalinergic neurones close to the raphe nucleus in the PAG; just how these two groups of cells are inter-related is unknown but it is reasonable to believe that they are both concerned with the suppression of pain through a descending pathway.

Endorphins in the control of pain

It has recently become known that electrical stimulation of the brain increases endorphin production, which results in a higher endorphin level in the cerebrospinal fluid withdrawn from the lumbar region. At the Centre for Pain Relief, Walton Hospital, Liverpool, tests are being made to determine whether there is an increased production of endogenous opiates following percutaneous cervical cordotomy and the pituitary injection of alcohol when these procedures relieve pain. One of the interesting features of neuromodulation of the brain is that, in most cases, withdrawal symptoms and/ or return of pain occurs following an injection of naloxone. Similar results are found on occasion following percutaneous cervical cordotomy and the injection of alcohol into the pituitary. There is no obvious correlation between pain relief and return of pain following the injection of naloxone in these patients, and work continues at the Centre for Pain Relief in Liverpool (Bowsher and Lipton, 1978, work in progress).

It is also known that pain relief obtained by acupuncture can be reversed by naloxone (Mayer, Price and Rafii, 1977). It would thus appear likely that all methods of pain relief are affected in some way by release of endogenous opiates; if the opiate antagonist naloxone is injected, pain relief is antagonized, causing the return of pain and, possibly, withdrawal symptoms.

References

Atweh, S. F. and Kuhar, M. J. (1977). Autoradiographic localisation of opiate receptors in rat brain. i. Spinal cord and lower medulla. *Brain Research*, **124**, 53–68; ii. The brain stem. **129**, 1–12; iii. The telencephalon. **134**, 393–406.

Elde, R., Hökfelt, T., Johansson, O. and Terenius, L. (1976). Immunohistochemical studies using antibodies to leucine-enkephalin: initial observations on the nervous system of the rat. *Neuroscience* **1**, 349–351.

Henry, J. L. (1975). Substance P excitation of spinal nociceptive neurones. *Neuroscience Abstracts* **1**, 390.

Henry, J. L. (1976). Effects of substance P on functionally identified units in cat spinal cord. *Brain Research* **114**, 439–451.

Hökfelt, T., Elde, R., Johansson, O., Luft, R., Nilsson, G. and Arimura, A. (1976). Immunohistochemical evidence for separate populations of somatostatin-containing and substance-P-containing primary afferent neurons in the rat. *Neuroscience* **1**, 131–136.

Hökfelt, T., Elde, R., Johansson, O., Terenius, L. and Stein, L. (1977). The distribution of enkephalin-immunoreactive cell bodies in the rat central nervous system. *Neuroscience Letters* **5**, 25–31.

Hosobuchi, Y., Adams, J. E. and Linchitz, R. (1977). Pain relief by electrical stimulation of the central grey matter in humans and its reversal by naloxone. *Science* **197**, 183–185.

Hughes, J., Smith, T. W., Kosterlitz, H. W., Fothergill, L. A., Morgan, B. A. and Morris, H. R. (1975). Identification of two related pentapeptides from the brain with potent opiate agonist activity. *Nature* **258**, 577–579.

Jessell, T. M. and Iversen, L. L. (1977). Opiate analgesics inhibit substance P release from rat trigeminal nucleus. *Nature* **268**, 549–551.

Mayer, D. J., Price, D. D. and Rafii, A. (1977). Antagonism of acupuncture analgesia in man by the narcotic antagonist naloxone. *Brain Research* **121**, 368–372.

Mayer, D. J., Wolfe, T. L., Akil, H., Carder, B. and Liebeskind, J. C. (1971). Analgesia from electrical stimulation in the brain-stem of the rat. *Science* **174**, 1351–1354.

Miles, J. B. (1978). Personal communication.

Pert, C. B. and Snyder, S. H. (1973). Opiate receptor: demonstration in nervous tissue. *Science* **179**, 1011–1014.

Pert, C. B. and Yaksh, T. L. (1974). Sites of morphine-induced analgesia in the primate brain: relation to pain pathways. *Brain Research* **80**, 135–140.

Proudfitt, H. K. and Anderson, E. G. (1975). Morphine analgesia: blockade by raphe magnus lesions. *Brain Research* **98**, 612–618.

Richardson, D. E. and Akil, H. (1977). Pain reduction by electrical brain stimulation in man. 1. Acute administration in periaqueductal and periventricular sites. *Journal of Neurosurgery* **47**, 178–183; 2. Chronic self-administration in the periventricular grey matter. **47**, 184–194.

Simantov, R., Showman, A. M. and Snyder, S. H. (1976). A morphine-like factor enkephalin in rat brain: subcellular localization. *Brain Research* **107**, 650–657.

Simantov, R., Kuhar, M. J., Pasternak, G. W. and Snyder, S. H. (1976). The regional distribution of a morphine-like factor enkephalin in monkey brain. *Brain Research* **106**, 189–197.

Simon, E. J., Hiller, J. M. and Edelman, I. (1973). Stereospecific binding of the potent narcotic analgesic ^{3}H-etorphine to rat brain homogenate. *Proceedings of the National Academy of Sciences, U.S.A.* **70**, 1947–1949.

Snyder, S. H. (1977). Opiate receptors and internal opiates. *Scientific American* **236**, 44–56.

Terenius, L. (1973). Stereospecific interaction between narcotic analgesics and a synaptic plasma membrane fraction of rat cerebral cortex. *Acta Pharmacologica et Toxicologica* **32**, 317–320.

Vale, W., Brazeau, P., Rivier, C., Brown, M., Boss, B., Rivier, J., Burgus, R., Ling, N. and Guilleman, R. (1975). Somatostatin. *Recent Progress in Hormone Research* **31**, 365–392.

von Euler, U. S. and Gaddum, H. J. (1931). An unidentified depressor substance in certain tissue extracts. *Journal of Physiology* **72**, 74–87.

5

Varieties of pain

Sensations such as touch, sight and hearing have a quantitative relationship with the stimulus producing them. This is not the case with pain, which is a private experience appreciated when a tissue-damaging stimulus is applied to the peripheral tissues. This private experience involves an element of suffering.

Two types of pain can be appreciated. Pricking pain, called first pain, is accurately located, is felt only in skin, is rapidly conducted and is not prolonged. It is carried by spinothalamic fibres. Second pain is felt in skin or in deep tissues. It is diffuse, poorly localized, conducts slowly and is prolonged (i.e. it outlasts the stimulus provoking it). It is carried by spinoreticular fibres. When second pain develops and does not disappear, it becomes pathological pain.

Broadly speaking, pathological pain can be divided into four groups:

(1) Superficial pain.
(2) Deep pain.
(3) Neurological pain.
(4) Psychological pain.

Each of these has its own characteristics but they all have features in common. A pathological pain is always accompanied by an alteration or disturbance of mood, which is related to an element of suffering. In addition, there are associated elements of fear, depression, anxiety or agitation.

Pain persists for as long as the stimulus producing it is present and it does not adapt; the alterations of mood produced by pathological pain do not adapt but they may deepen and become more marked.

The flexor reflex is a protective reflex causing automatic withdrawal of a limb from a dangerous situation. Similar reflexes come into play when a joint is damaged or a tissue is inflamed, producing, for example, the abdominal rigidity of peritonitis. There are, in addition, other effects such as the protection of the affected part and the cessation of activity. Lesser degrees of damage alter this picture to varying degree. Corresponding autonomic responses occur which include changes in blood pressure, sweating, nausea and vomiting. These reflex and autonomic changes persist while pathological pain is present and, although some are more marked than others, some may persist after the original injury has disappeared.

Superficial and deep pain do not require much discussion but neurological pain is of great interest to clinicians and three types are mentioned in some detail: phantom limb, causalgia and post-herpetic neuralgia. Following this, a brief mention is made of some types of psychological pain and the conditions which produce it.

Superficial pain

Superficial pain is sharp, light and well localized, and there is muscular activity.

Deep pain

Deep pain, on the contrary, is aching, dull and not localized, and there is decreased muscular activity. On occasion, the pain is referred not to its origin but to some other related area (Kellgren, 1939), as when irritation of the central portion of the diaphragm is referred to the shoulder or peripheral diaphragmatic irritation is referred to the lower thoracic region. Not only is the pain referred but often there is also an area of hyperaesthesia in the referred area and sometimes the pain is relieved by a local injection of anaesthetic solutions into the hyperaesthetic area. The explanation of this phenomenon is that facilitation in the spinal cord produces the hyperaesthesia, and a reduction of sensory input will reduce the segmental cord activity and decrease the facilitation.

Neurological pain

Neurological pain arises from lesions of the c.n.s. central to the sensory nerve endings. The pain has an intense, unpleasant burning sensation which is diffuse, poorly localized and often prolonged. There are two varieties of pain: one, called hyperalgesia, in which the threshold is lowered; and one, hyperpathia, where the threshold is raised.

These pains are influenced by mood and emotional state and may be triggered by stimuli not normally regarded as painful. Thus, the slight stimulus from the wind blowing over the skin, or the normal rubbing of clothes against the skin, may be sufficient to initiate the peculiarly unpleasant pain.

Phantom limb pain

This type of neurological pain arises after a limb has been excised. The amputation sections nerves, and when these regenerate they form a terminal neuroma containing many fine partially regenerated nerve fibres. These fine nerve endings are peculiarly sensitive to vibration or pressure (Wall and Gutnick, 1974).

There is the possibility that pain in the limb before amputation engrams a portion of the c.n.s. so that this responds to peripheral stimulation after amputation with a similar pain response to that felt before the amputation. Many patients who have had amputations continue to feel the same pain post-amputation that they felt pre-amputation and it may be accurately localized to exactly the same place in the phantom limb.

All patients who have amputations feel the presence of a phantom which is usually non-painful although there may be mild tingling in it for a while. These eventually die away and the phantom also disappears from consciousness; however, if pain remains, the painful phantom does not disappear. It is not only amputations of limbs which produce painful phantoms; any amputated part does so—there are well authenticated cases of phantom breasts following mastectomy.

Types of phantom limbs

The descriptions some patients give of their phantoms are so peculiar that one is tempted to believe that they are making up a story. Such is not the case. The pain does not always arise in a pre-existing phantom, as some patients have the usual post-amputation transient phantom which disappears and yet develop a painful phantom in later years. Some patients have no sense of connection between the painful phantom and the stump, so they may have a painful phantom foot suspended below the stump in a position corresponding to its normal place.

Most phantoms tend to shorten in time so that—to continue with the example of a painful foot—the foot feels as though it is attached to the end of the stump with no intervening leg, though some patients have a mini-leg in between. Some patients feel the phantom inside the stump so that the foot seems to be within the stump.

The position of the phantom can be bizarre and may remain in the same position, but many patients say that whatever the position of the phantom when they wake up each morning, so it remains all day. Others can move the phantom, or a portion of it, at will but often at the expense of an increase in pain. Occasionally the phantom is as freely movable as a normal limb.

At times there are problems when the patient wears an artificial limb as the phantom may be in a very different position to the artificial one. Some patients mention that the phantom takes up the position of the artificial one, or that a phantom hand which is in a shortened position will extend to that of the artificial one.

There are many more unusual features about phantom limbs which are too numerous to detail here.

Treatment

Treatment of phantom limb pain is difficult because, in many amputees, there are psychological alterations which must be treated. All patients who do not respond to the simpler methods of pain control should be assessed by a psychiatrist. As with cancer or vascular pain, patients suffering from phantom limb pain concentrate their whole attention on their pain; if they have had a series of pain treatments and have visited a number of specialist centres for this purpose without obtaining relief, the mental pressures on them are enormous.

Depression. Amputees may need treating for depression or anxiety, or both, and the presence of these is understandable. Amitriptyline is a very useful drug as it is an antidepressant with mild sedative action as well. There are uncomfortable side effects with this drug and it should be given at night in doses of 50 mg. The patient should be told that he must take it for at least ten days before its action becomes apparent.

Vibration. The simplest method of treating those with phantom limb pain is to use a vibrator on the painful portion of the stump. The small nerve fibrils which are sensitive to pressure degenerate if intermittent pressure is applied to them. The old technique of tapping the end of a painful stump with a small rubber hammer is well documented and works in some patients.

Neuroma. If the stump is palpated, it is sometimes possible to feel a fusiform tender area or, if it is not fusiform, a palpable, excruciatingly tender swelling. These are most likely due to the presence of a neuroma. The swollen region can be injected with local anaesthetic, such as 2 per cent lignocaine; this should be done as gently as possible because the mere insertion of a needle is very painful, while the injection into the solid material of the neuroma increases pressure in this tender structure. If a phantom limb is present as well as stump pain, the injection is likely to cause pain in the phantom. There may be more than one painful area in the stump and all will require injection.

If a neuroma is present and has been correctly injected, the pain will be relieved. A check can be made when the pain returns by using a longer acting local anaesthetic such as 0·5 per cent bupivacaine and observing if a longer period of pain relief occurs on this occasion. Finally, 6–8 per cent phenol in water can be injected after a small quantity of local anaesthetic to see if a really long-lasting result can be obtained.

Operation. If the presence of a neuroma has been demonstrated, it is reasonable to refer the patient to a surgeon for consideration of excision. Excision is no guarantee that the pain will be relieved completely, as in an appreciable number of patients the pain returns. Further excision may or may not provide a further period of pain relief.

Transcutaneous neuromodulation. This method often relieves the pain of stump and phantom limbs but it is essential that the electrodes are applied to residual nerve strands supplying the stump. This is somewhat simpler in the leg than in the arm as the sciatic nerve can be stimulated in the stump. When this method works it cannot always be used in everyday life because the electrodes may not be maintained easily in position (Campbell and Long, 1976).

Dorsal column stimulation (*DCS*). When other methods have been tried and failed, the possibility of dorsal column stimulation should be considered. Various tests, including those already mentioned, can be carried out to predict the likely efficacy of DCS.

Nerve abrasion. This is the name given to stimulation of the residual nerve strands in or near the stump. If the manœuvre does not produce pain or reproduce the pain complained of, then it must be assumed that the central connections of the peripheral nerves are incomplete. This means that for any DCS to be effective it must be performed at a higher level. This type of injury frequently occurs following distraction injuries of the brachial plexus from motor cycle accidents. It results in the brachial plexus being torn from the spinal cord, with injury to the arm which may necessitate amputation (Nashold, Wilson and Slaughter, 1969; Nashold and Friedman, 1972).

Acupuncture. Acupuncture should be considered as another form of peripheral nerve stimulation; if it relieves the pain, it can be regarded as corroborative evidence that stimulation methods will work. The acupuncture needles are inserted in dermatomal distribution; the actual positions are not particularly important except that they must be placed in an area of skin with normal sensation. Acupuncture is considered in detail in Chapter 12.

Hypertonic saline. Another form of peripheral stimulation, hypertonic saline also provides additional evidence as to the likely effectiveness of stimulation methods in the treatment of the patient. The strength of saline used is 7·5 per cent. Not more than 1·0 ml is injected into the interspinous ligament at the dermatomal level of the pain. Injection to one or other side of the ligament will refer intense pain locally to the side injected. If the interspinous ligament is injected, the pain is referred to a central position but may be referred to the painful side only. After a few minutes during which pain in the stump or phantom increases enormously, it dies out. The patient then has a period of discomfort in an interspinous position but no pain in the stump or phantom.

As mentioned previously, when all or at least the majority of these tests are positive, a DC epidural stimulation test can be carried out by means of a temporary implant.

Causalgia

Causalgia is another variety of neurological pain, classically occurring on a battlefield when a bullet passes close to, but does not sever, a nerve trunk. The pain may occur immediately or as long as one year later. It is a most unpleasant pain which is burning in type, spreads diffusely and is aggravated by the slightest movement or touch on the affected part. The pain is excruciating and the patient adopts a typical posture and attitude which protects the part from touch, vibration or movement. Trophic changes occur, including osteoporosis, muscle atrophy and a changed appearance of the skin which becomes red and shiny (de Takats, 1945).

Civilian injuries following accident or operation can produce the syndrome described above but usually to a lesser degree. The complete syndrome is often known as a 'major reflex dystrophy,' while lesser varieties are called 'minor reflex dystrophies'. An example of the minor variety would be Sudeck's atrophy which has been mentioned already.

Another reflex dystrophy commonly seen is the 'shoulder–hand syndrome' or 'frozen shoulder' in which a painful shoulder is combined with oedema of the hand, although either may predominate. It often occurs after a myocardial infarction or after an injury to the shoulder.

All these dystrophies should be treated by sympathetic block. Sometimes a single block is sufficient to produce permanent benefit but in most cases the procedure has to be repeated a number of times. As long as there is an increasing benefit each time the block is performed, then it is worth while continuing with them. If the period of relief is only a little longer than the action of the local anaesthetic agent used, then it will be necessary to try to achieve sympathetic block by other methods such as the use of intravenous guanethidine (Hannington-Kiff, 1974).

In the upper arm a diagnostic stellate ganglion block is easily carried out. The basis of the technique is that the sympathetic ganglia in the neck, including the stellate ganglion which lies on the neck of the first rib, lie anterior to the prevertebral fascia. Thus if local anaesthetic solutions are deposited on this fascia higher up in the neck and the patient's head is raised slightly, the solution will diffuse downwards covering the sympathetic fibres and rapidly reaching the stellate ganglion. All that is necessary is to insert a 21 gauge needle medial to the carotid artery until it hits the anterior border of one of the transverse processes. A slight withdrawal will then place the tip anterior to the prevertebral fascia and the anaesthetic solution can be injected. Sometimes the solution spreads in part on to the somatic nerves in this region, producing some weakness of the upper limb, or to the recurrent laryngeal nerve, producing transient husky voice.

All the patients will develop a Horner's syndrome—ptosis, miosis, enophthalmos, anhydrosis and vasodilatation—but this is not certain evidence that sympathetic fibres to the arm and hand have been affected. The upper limb is supplied from the four or five upper thoracic segments and not all sympathetic fibres to the upper limb pass through the stellate ganglion. It is never wise to make a decision on sympathectomy by a stellate ganglion block alone. A positive effect can be accepted but not a negative one unless either paravertebral blocks to the upper four dorsal spinal nerves or the intravenous guanethidine method have been used as well.

Guanethidine sympathetic block

This useful method was advocated by Hannington-Kiff (1974). Some 10–15 mg guanethidine (Ismelin) is used for the upper limb, and 15–25 mg for the lower. An indwelling intravenous needle is inserted into any convenient arm or leg vein and fixed in position. The limb is then raised to drain it of venous blood. A sphygmomanometer cuff is inflated above systolic pressure, and the guanethidine with 500 units of heparin made up to 20–30 ml of solution with 0·5 per cent lignocaine is injected. The cuff is kept inflated for 20 minutes or so and then carefully deflated incrementally, monitoring the blood pressure during this period in case some of the guanethidine escapes into the general circulation, producing a hypotension. A sympathetic block of a limb produced in this fashion will last at least one week.

Lumbar sympathetic block

This is a very useful and simple block to carry out if an image intensifier is available. If an image intensifier is not used, then the block can be carried out by the classical method in which the needle impinges on the side of the lumbar vertebra and then is gradually moved anteriorly until the needle slides past it.

With an image intensifier the same technique is much easier, as the transverse process of the lumbar vertebrae can be seen and avoided, and the needle tip is placed quickly and accurately anterolaterally on the vertebra in close proximity to the lumbar sympathetic chain. If only one injection is to be made then the chain is injected at L2, when it is said to diffuse widely over the whole chain. This often does happen and to make sure that all the lumbar sympathetic fibres are affected the author believes that three needles must be used, at L2, L3 and L4. The needles are placed in position and electrical skin thermometers are placed on the thighs, calves and feet in corresponding positions on the two sides, the normal limb acting as a control for the one being blocked. The legs must not be covered and the temperature of the two limbs is allowed to reach equilibrium (while this is going on the needles can be inserted). Lignocaine (5 ml 2 per cent) is injected through the upper needle and the temperature monitored for five minutes. Another 5 ml is then injected at L3 and the temperature is monitored for a further five minutes; the same process is repeated at L4. Although the maximum rise in normal legs is found after the L2 injection, there will be slight additional rises in temperature after each of the others. In other words, the lumbar sympathetic nerves are to some extent segmented and this is important if a diagnostic trial for sympathectomy is being carried out. Personal experience has shown that when the foot is affected—say by a threatened gangrene from vascular insufficiency, or from a causalgia—blocking L4 may have a relatively greater effect than a block of the other segments. It is of value for this effect alone. The procedure is time consuming but it is usually effective.

Post-herpetic neuralgia

The developed condition of post-herpetic neuralgia is the most difficult to treat of all those painful conditions regularly referred to a centre for pain relief. The time when it is easiest to help the herpetic patient is before the condition becomes established. After post-herpetic neuralgia has developed, usually the most that can be done is to reduce the pain. A few patients obtain complete relief of pain when treated at a late stage but most do not obtain significant pain relief, and the expectations of patient and physician should not be high. Herpes zoster is an acute viral infection affecting the posterior spinal root ganglion and the spinal nerves of the corresponding ganglia of the cranial nerves. The virus appears in chickenpox (varicella) and is of the DNA type. It is believed that, once infected in childhood, the virus lies dormant in adults until the immunity falls, when it replicates again and the disease tends to be confined to a local distribution as immunity quickly rises; this accounts for the local segmental distribution of the manifestations. The infection is probably initiated by trauma or infection, and the presence of hidden malignancy should be considered. The disease commonly affects the thoracic spinal nerves. The first division of the trigeminal nerve is the branch most often affected of cranial nerves. This is due to the fact that, anatomically, the first division descends lowest in the spinal cord.

The skin eruptions occur on the third or fourth day when the skin is reddened and vesicles appear. They dry up in five or six days, leaving small scars which sometimes become confluent but on occasion no scars result. It is believed that ganglionitis in the posterior root ganglion produces an autonomic imbalance and the skin eruption is due to this; an alternative theory is that the virus passes along the peripheral nerves antidromically. The pain of the acute stage disappears as the vesicles heal but, especially in old people, may continue for years though there is a tendency in the milder cases for the condition to settle. Treatment of the chronic condition stands the best chance of succeeding before three months; after six months, it is rarely completely relieved by simple treatments.

The infection may not remain in the posterior root ganglion and posterior horn but can spread into the anterior horn, producing paresis. Indeed there can be spread into the bulbar region or even into the brain, producing an encephalitis. These latter conditions can occur with any virus infection.

In the older patients pain, dysaesthesiae and hyperaesthesiae continue after the acute phase and these are all increased by minor stimuli. In some patients it is not the pain which is disturbing but the accompanying discomfort. Thus there are two elements to the chronic condition, the relative amount of each varying with the individual but in any case the pain has a peculiarly unpleasant character to it similar to that which occurs in the dystrophies.

In the acute herpes zoster infection there is selective destruction of nerve fibres because of a tendency for proportionately more of the larger nerve fibres to be destroyed than of the smaller ones, and when regeneration of the large fibres occurs they tend to have smaller diameters than before the infection. In addition, there is a relative loss of large fibres with age. In this way after a zoster infection the population of nerve fibres in the skin tends to shift in the direction of fewer large ones and more small ones; on gate control theory a change in this direction tends to keep the gate open so that painful stimuli pass more easily.

Treatment

Prevention of the disease is the best way of treating it, and idoxuridine (Herpid) inhibits a proportion of cases with DNA virus infections. The treatment begins as soon as the diagnosis is certain—usually as soon as the rash appears. Idoxuridine is painted on four times per day for four days. This treatment can be instituted by the general practitioner. Another method of treatment is to use steroids either topically on the rash or in massive doses systemically but the disadvantage of this drug is that occasionally widespread dissemination of the disease results. The use of steroids is said to reduce the incidence of post-herpetic neuralgia but the claims do not seem to be generally recognized (Editorial, 1976).

There is a third method of treatment in the acute phase: by systemic and sympathetic nerve blocks (Colding, 1967, 1969, 1973); after sympathetic block of the affected region, the pain and vesiculation can be reduced. Whether the fact that the patient does not develop post-herpetic neuralgia is a result of the sympathetic block cannot be proved, as the majority of patients who have a zoster infection do not develop chronic pain.

Probably the best treatment is to use idoxuridine because this will heal the vesicles as well as reducing the pain in about three-quarters of the patients. Unfortunately, even after this treatment, some patients will undoubtedly develop chronic pain.

Chronic pain is the complaint with which the patient visits a pain relief clinic and, as there is no certain method to relieve their pain and discomfort, it is necessary to have a scheme of treatment available and to work through it steadily. It is important for the patient to accept the idea, before treatment, that his pain is due to a mild type of nerve damage which occurred during the infection, and that it is unlikely that this can be repaired so that he obtains complete relief. Nevertheless, it may be possible to find a treatment which will help such patients so that pain is reduced. They are informed that there is no way of knowing which particular treatment will help, and so they must give each method a fair trial.

The simplest of all methods is to try peripheral nerve stimulation; as the condition is due to an imbalance of peripheral nerve action, it is logical to see if either transcutaneous neuromodulation or acupuncture will help. If transcutaneous stimulation is used, then provision should be made for the patient to have the stimulator at home over a period of several months, provided that the initial test gave benefit. In many patients electrical stimulation merely increases the discomfort and pain and has to be stopped (Nathan and Wall, 1974).

Acupuncture is used dermatomally or through the classical acupuncture points for the area and type of disease if these are known. Ideally, a daily gentle session should be carried out but as it is impossible to carry out acupuncture this often in clinic practice, a lesser frequency must be used—either once a week or, if this is impracticable, once every two weeks. The acupuncture needles must not be placed in anaesthetic areas, and if these are extensive the needles may be positioned at the same dermatomal level on the normal side.

Any neurological pain tends to have a psychological element to it; for this reason it is worth trying the effect of psychotropic drugs. The combination of a substituted phenothiazine with a tricyclic antidepressant is commonly used and may help (Taub and Collins, 1974), particularly in depressed patients who are usually living on their own. Fluphenazine 4 mg per day and amitriptyline up to 75 mg at night should be tried for one month. It has not proved of general value in our practice though the occasional patient is helped. A trial of the 'cold spray' which is a mixture of trichlorofluoromethane 85 per cent in dichlorodifluoromethane 15 per cent in a spray can (PR Spray) is innocuous and is well worth a trial as even when it fails to provide continuous relief (as it usually does) it does help to ease exacerbations of the pain first thing in the morning or for getting off to sleep. It must be used correctly by 'washing' the fluid over the whole of the painful region, waiting one minute to avoid a frostbite, and then repeating the 'wash' and the wait twice more. This procedure is repeated whenever the pain returns to its previous level over the first two days, and when beneficial, the period between each 'wash' is gradually extended so that in the most satisfactory cases the patient only has to use it three or four times per day. Spray cans are used up rapidly so the patient must have a good supply—six or seven at a time.

Subcutaneous injections of local anaesthetic (0·5 per cent lignocaine) are tried first, and if these fail or only partly succeed, a long-acting steroid such as methylprednisolone acetate (Depo-Medrone) is added. These solutions may be injected weekly, fortnightly or monthly as required and do seem to have some effect on the hyperpathia and dysaesthesiae.

A careful watch must be kept on the total amount of methylprednisolone acetate used as Cushing's syndrome may develop. Following this injection nerve blocks can be tried, the most satisfactory being those of purely or mainly sensory nerves such as the intercostals or branches of the trigeminal nerve. If simple diagnostic blocks succeed on a number of occasions, carried out to avoid placebo reactions, then long-acting blocks can be considered. One word of warning as far as the trigeminal nerve is concerned: blocking of branches seems to be effective on occasion but permanent block of the gasserian ganglion itself is dangerous because, after a short initial period of relief, the pain usually returns and is even worse than before. Our experience with this type of interference is not satisfactory.

Subarachnoid phenol blocks relieve the pain but not the dysaesthesiae and patients will complain bitterly if this is not explained carefully to them beforehand. This is why the subarachnoid block is not used at the Liverpool Centre for Pain Relief and the most central of the injections used is made paravertebrally. Sympathetic blocks can be tried and will sometimes relieve some of the discomfort and pain but not to the extent they do in the acute stage.

If the above simple methods do not help, more complicated neurosurgical procedures are available. Such procedures as cordotomy are unwise, partly because they may not relieve the pain even when a complete and satisfactory analgesic level has been produced, but mainly because these patients have a normal expectation of life and cordotomies wear off in time.

Percutaneous electrical stimulation is the only remaining method which offers any prospect of regular success, and a temporary epidural stimulator implant can be tried with only a little increased hazard to the patient.

Psychological pain

All patients who become ill show changes in their personality and while these changes are minimal during short illness where discomfort, pain and personal disability can be withstood because the end result is near and the benefit is obvious and certain, patients with chronic conditions are in a very different situation and the way they cope with the stress of illness depends on their personality. The prospect of a chronic painful condition, further major surgery and, ultimately, death is enough to affect the strongest personality.

Naturally, everyone who becomes ill becomes anxious; however, some patients who are normally anxious develop tension of such degree that it may need treatment in its own right. Furthermore, anxiety increases the appreciation of pain, and also produces variations to the pain level depending on the emotional state so that it is insufficient to treat a patient's pain without treating his anxiety also. Other patients are easily depressed and problems are seen in a pessimistic fashion which is shown by depression. Such patients feel pain more severely than those with an optimistic personality and they tend to concentrate on aspects of illness relating to suffering and death.

It must be remembered that pain often occurs as a symptom in mental illness, especially in the depressive type, and it is believed that this is a mechanism by which intolerable mental pressures are transferred to physical suffering which then can be dealt with more easily by the depressed person. If the pain completely hides the mental depression, the depression is said to be masked, but often depression and pain are present together.

Some patients become preoccupied with their normal bodily feelings and functions and the slightest variation brings on worries about the cause. Minor aches and pains are common in daily life but the reaction of these patients to the common stresses is quite inappropriate. They often have a long history of worries about minor conditions and they may copy the illness of a close relative or friend. This is the condition of hypochondriasis which can be a mental disorder or part of an anxiety or hysterical neurosis. It also occurs in depressive illnesses and in schizophrenia.

Hysterics show immature behaviour and immature emotions, and develop highly emotional situations which exhaust everybody except the hysteric. When these patients suffer pain, the normal tendency to exaggeration becomes obvious with their use of highly descriptive phrases and dramatic gestures. They do not suffer pain easily and care has to be taken that, while suspicious of their exaggeration, the physician does not miss the underlying physical cause.

Obsessional patients need regularity in life. They cannot stand uncertainty and this means that the treatment of painful physical illness is difficult. They constantly want more information about their illness, its cause, the possible future and the various treatments than any doctor can give. The slightest hesitation by the doctor is seized upon, and the best way of dealing with this type of patient is to be absolutely truthful and concise. A difficult prospect.

So far, mention has been made of those mental variations which, when carried to excess, become psychoses. However, most human beings have a tendency to one or other of these varieties and there are circumstances in which the patient uses his pain—either consciously or unconsciously—to manipulate his surroundings and his relatives.

Operant conditioning

From the above it will be seen that pain can be real (i.e. organic) though modified by the individual psychological attitude; or it can be imaginary and a reflection of a psychogenic disease. To believe that imaginary pain is non-existent is quite unrealistic and does not help treatment. Whether pain is produced from a real or an imaginary cause, it is still very real to the patient. However, some patients use a chronic condition to control their environment. Most of these patients have pain and are limited in their activity and may be bed-ridden. They do not usually have well adjusted personalities and are frequently unsuccessful. Their lives centre on their pain and, as no human activity is free of motive, it must be asked 'what motive have these patients, what reward do they get for living in this invalid style?'

The answer is to be found in what is called 'operant conditioning'. Life is a series of actions and reactions (Berne, 1964) and if there is a reward or some satisfaction following an action, then that action will be repeated to produce the satisfactory reaction once again. A behavioural pattern develops in this way, and conditioning of this type—the alteration of behaviour by a reward—is known as operant conditioning.

An unsuccessful, anxious, dissatisfied person, shunned and avoided by his fellows may find that during an illness more pleasant responses arise from those around him. A painful condition will produce attention and pleasant treatment, much more than he normally receives. Not only that, but the patient is relieved of making any difficult decision such as going to work and earning a living, or having to face up to what may be an unpleasant and difficult life.

Such a patient can opt to allow the situation to stay at this level. He adopts, consciously or unconsciously, the career of being a patient in pain and is not concerned with obtaining relief (Szasz, 1968). Obviously if operant conditioning produces this type of patient, then operant conditioning by suitable arrangement of the environment should be able to reverse it. The basis of operant conditioning to modify pain behaviour is for the doctors, nurses and relatives to ignore the patient's complaint of pain in such a way as not to reinforce it. Any analgesics administered are given regularly and in sufficient quantity so that obtaining these drugs is not dependent upon the patient expressing pain and thus they are given at a fixed time whether pain is present or not (Fordyce *et al.*, 1973; Greenhoot and Sternbach, 1974). For instance, if the patient looks pale and unhappy and moans, no notice is taken of him under operant conditioning treatment. To take notice, offer sympathy and hand out drugs will reinforce the operant that the patient is using—namely, looking and sounding uncomfortable. Only when the patient becomes active and helpful is notice taken. In this way the desired type of behaviour is reinforced with attention. One of the most potent operants is the doctor prescribing drugs as needed. In other words, if pain is present, give the drugs; thus if no pain is present, there are no drugs, and one cannot blame the patient under these circumstances for exaggerating pain behaviour. Operant reconditioning involves not just carrying out the above technical procedure but also bringing the patient's family, work-mates and the patient himself into the procedure by explaining and showing what is being done. Also, the patient has to be removed from his normal environment so that control can be obtained over the operants.

The operant reconditioning team must be specially trained because the idea of being unsympathetic to a patient in pain is foreign to doctors and nurses, which is why one of the most important factors (both for the staff and for the patient) is to know that adequate medication is being given. The patient is also told that at some stage during his reconditioning the amount of analgesic in his medication will be reduced. The medication is given in a fluid form with a heavily masking taste and colour. Thus, the patient cannot judge from the colour or the taste what quantity of analgesics he is receiving although he does know that, in the initial stages, the dose of analgesics will be at least as much as he has been receiving outside.

During reconditioning, the patient keeps a record of daily activity because the whole purpose of the reconditioning is to bring the patient into increased social activity. Comments by the ward staff on these records are invaluable by praising progress and making suggestions if the expected results are slow in coming. Some workers using the operant conditioning method also use group treatment sessions. In this way there is a positive feedback to the patient from the staff and other patients. In fact, one of the most beneficial arrangements is for other patients in similar circumstances of operant reconditioning to comment on their fellows. Usually they cannot be fooled as they themselves have been using all the gambits available from the advantages of having a painful condition. They are never backward in pointing out the tricks their fellows get up to.

References

Berne, E. (1964). *The Games People Play*. Penguin, Harmondsworth.
Campbell, J. N. and Long, D. M. (1976). Peripheral nerve stimulation in the treatment of intractable pain. *Journal of Neurosurgery* **45,** 692–699.
Colding, A. (1967). Regional block in acute herpes zoster. *Der Anaesthesist* **16,** 172.
Colding, A. (1969). Effect of regional sympathetic blocks in the treatment of herpes zoster. *Acta Anaesthesiologica Scandinavica* **13,** 133–141.
Colding, A. (1973). Treatment of acute herpes zoster. *Proceedings of the Royal Society of Medicine* **66,** 541–543.
de Takats, G. (1945). Causalgia states in peace and war. *Journal of the American Medical Association. 128,* 699.
Editorial (1976). Chemotherapy for varicella-zoster infections. *British Medical Journal* **2,** 1466–1467.
Fordyce, W. E., Fowler, R. S., Lehmann, J. F., De Latour, B. J., Sand, P. L. and Trieschmann, R. B. (1973). Operant conditioning in the treatment of chronic pain. *Archives of Physical Medicine and Rehabilitation* **54,** 399.
Greenhoot, J. A. and Sternbach, R. A. (1974). Varieties of pain games. In: *Advances in Neurology*, Vol. 4, pp. 598–9. Ed. by J. J. Bonica. Raven Press, New York.

Hannington-Kiff, J. G. (Ed.) (1974). Intravenous regional sympathetic block. In: *Pain Relief*, p. 69. Heinemann Medical, London.

Kellgren, J. H. (1939). On the distribution of pain arising from deep somatic structures with charts of segmental pain areas. *Clinical Science* **4**, 35.

Nashold, B. S. and Friedman, H. (1972). Dorsal column stimulation for the control of pain. Preliminary report of 30 cases. *Journal of Neurosurgery* **36**, 590–597.

Nashold, B. S., Wilson, W. P. and Slaughter, D. G. (1969). Stereotactic midbrain lesions for central dysaesthesia and phantom limb pain. Preliminary report. *Journal of Neurosurgery* **30**, 116–126.

Nathan P. W. and Wall P. D. (1974) Treatment of post-herpetic neuralgia by prolonged electric stimulation. *British Medical Journal* **3**, 645–647.

Szasz, T. S. (1968). The psychology of persistent pain: a portrait of l'homme douloureux. In: *Pain*. Ed. by A. Soulairac, J. Cahn and J. Charpentier. Academic Press, New York.

Taub, A. and Collins, W. F. (1974). Observations on the treatment of denervation dysesthesia with psychotropic drugs: postherpetic neuralgia, anesthesia dolorosa, peripheral neuropathy. In: *Advances in Neurology*, Vol. 4, pp. 309–315. Ed. by J. J. Bonica. Raven Press, New York.

Wall, P. D. and Gutnick, M. (1974). Properties of afferent nerve impulses originating from a neuroma. *Nature*, **248**, 740–743.

Further reading

Berne, E. (1964). *The Games People Play*. Penguin, Harmondsworth.

Merskey, H. (1977). Psychiatric management of patients with chronic pain. In: *Persistent Pain*, p. 113. Ed. by S. Lipton. Academic Press, London and New York.

Sternbach, R. A. (1974). *Pain Patients: traits and treatment*. Academic Press, New York and London.

6
Pain relief clinics

There are a number of types of pain relief clinic and the boundary of one variety merges into another, but three basic types can be distinguished. There is the single-handed practice where a doctor interested in pain relief work sees a small number of patients from time to time without being organized for this work beyond the ability to carry out examinations and simple blocking procedures. Very often this consultant carries out the pain relief programme in between his normal work which may be any variety of consultant practice. In Britain this type of practice is normally carried out by anaesthetists and often makes use of time available between and after other consultant clinics. The number of patients seen in this way is limited, as are the facilities available; nevertheless, patients who have chronic pain problems can be seen and dealt with provided their condition requires only the simpler procedures.

At the other end of the scale is the multidisciplinary clinic in which a large number of different consultants are involved and will certainly include a physician, surgeon, neurologist, neurosurgeon, psychiatrist and anaesthetist. There will be a properly organized outpatient clinic with all that this entails in the way of junior medical help, proper nursing staff and the usual clerical and other ancillary help. There will be facilities for radiology. Initially, the patient is seen by one member of the large staff, having being allocated by the chairman or director of the unit to the consultant most likely to help him on first referral. This doctor will then assess the patient and draw up a scheme of investigation or diagnostic treatment if this is indicated. If the problem requires the opinion of other doctors, then this is arranged. Most patients do not require complicated assessments and treatments, and usually the initial referring doctor can deal with his patient. However, in those patients who have difficult problems, often of long standing, a joint opinion from the entire group may be necessary and there are arrangements for this once or perhaps twice a week when a number of the consultants meet and discuss the difficult pain problems. Before this happens the patient has been 'worked up' properly so that the results of any investigations and all the relevant background information are available to the multidisciplinary committee. Combined with this type of organization will be the training of post-graduates and also the integration of medical students in their undergraduate training. There is usually a proper rotation system for junior staff at different levels of their training programme to take part in the work of the multidisciplinary pain relief clinic.

It is obvious that there is a large gap between the single-handed type of practice and the multidisciplinary one, and in most cases an intermediate type of practice is carried out. In this there are outpatient facilities, arrangements for investigations, beds and operating room time. In this unit one or two doctors work together, with arrangements that other consultants can be called in when required; this is not carried out on a committee basis, the patient being referred in the usual outpatient fashion from one consultant to another.

A number of problems have arisen with the multidisciplinary system; the arrangements for the initial assessment and treatment of the patient are usually successful but in the arrangements for joint consultations difficulties arise. Normally, it is very difficult to get more than two consultants together at any one time and when the system involves five or six coming together on a regular basis the problems tend to become unsurmountable. One or other of the team gets held up by other work. In addition, it is usual that, for any given patient, the majority of the specialists present have nothing to add to the treatment and there is no need to see the patient. Their time is wasted, except in so far as they can see an interesting condition or join in the discussion. However, there is one occasion when it works well and that is as part of a teaching programme for medical and nursing staff. It seems to me that the best use of medical and other manpower can be made by developing along the lines of an intermediate clinic. In the case of the Centre for Pain Relief in Walton Hospital, Liverpool, this involves seven active clinicians in pain relief work. Four of these spend most of their time on pain relief work alone, while the other three are concerned in pain problems arising in their own disciplines. Naturally, all the facilities and all the consultants of the hospital are available for all patients when required.

The conditions treated by these various types of pain relief clinic arise in patients who have suffered chronic pain for more than a few months. It does not have to be particularly severe to merit referral although patients with very severe pain due to advanced cancer or phantom limb or severe post-herpetic neuralgia form about 30 per cent of those treated. There are rarely emergencies of pain in pain clinic work, the most likely one being an acute trigeminal neuralgia and this can usually be dealt with by means of carbamazepine (Tegretol). The only danger is that a patient with very severe pain may commit suicide but this is extremely rare and generally patients with chronic painful conditions do not die of their pain. However, it must be recognized that the mental makeup of patients with chronic painful conditions is such that they will rest content, or as near content as they can get, as long as they think nothing can be done about their pain but, as soon as they realize there is a clinic or a doctor who is able to help, they require instant treatment and the organization of the clinic should be cognizant of this.

Initially, the fashion in which patients are seen by the doctors of the pain relief centre has to be decided. It will depend to some extent on the normal practice in the country concerned but in Britain the pain relief clinic will, in most cases, be an internal referral clinic; that is, it will depend for its patients on the other specialist clinics in its own hospital and in the surrounding hospitals. This means that patients who are referred to the clinic have been seen and thoroughly investigated in the previous year either in hospital or in a hospital outpatient department. Most pain relief clinics are not equipped with staff to deal with all the general conditions which produce pain. The type of patient seen at a pain relief clinic has a chronic painful condition; it is not the purpose of a pain relief clinic to act as another general surgical or medical outpatient department. With these criteria it is possible to admit a patient direct from a general practitioner if the patient has been examined reasonably recently. Occasionally, a patient without this background is taken into the unit direct if the diagnosis is obvious, as in post-herpetic neuralgia where there is no point in burdening another clinic with this patient.

The diagnostic facilities available to a pain relief clinic will naturally depend on its size but in a fairly busy clinic one would expect there to be satisfactory outpatient facilities, involving the use of more than one room, and that in these rooms minor injection procedures can be carried out. The usual radiology of skull and skeleton should be available and, if necessary, facilities for procedures such as a metrizamide myelogram, e.c.g., e.m.g. and e.e.g., lung function tests and haematological investigations should also be present.

Ideally, there should be facilities available in the operating theatre for all the specialized techniques of pain relief. These may not all be performed by the same physician but certainly percutaneous cervical cordotomy and the transnasal, trans-sphenoidal injection of alcohol into the pituitary fossa should be possible. This means that an image intensifier is necessary and this must either belong to the centre for pain relief or be available with certainty on the operating day. Suitable nursing and ancillary help will be required in both outpatient and operating theatre areas, and one must take great care in the organization of such work that sufficient help is available as the tendency is to provide room and space but not enough people to run the space effectively. Just as much care and attention need to be paid to pain relief work in the outpatient department and operating theatre as with any other clinic.

A few words on the space required in the outpatient department are indicated, as this subject is often neglected. It should be satisfactory for its purpose. The examination couch should have enough space round it so that the examining doctor can stand on either side of the patient but, if this is not possible, there should be enough room for the couch to be pulled away from the wall when necessary. It is fairly easy to work out how much space is required when, for instance, an examination couch requires 15 square metres, two trolleys 9 square metres, storage cupboards about 11, desk and chairs about 13. In addition to this, a working space of about 1 metre all round the examination couch and about 0·6 metre round the desk, while a portable surgical lamp, filing cabinet, wash bowl and drug cupboard all require space. When this is added up, it is clear that the outpatient room should be between 4 and 4·5 metres square. The shape of the room can vary but working space around the patient is most important.

The equipment kept in the outpatient clinic will, of necessity, depend on the space available but wall charts do not take up any space and these can show the anatomy of relevant areas, particular types of blocks which may be used and other information to suit the taste or ability of the consultant and those he will train. Reference books nearby are required and ideally an image intensifier with a radiotranslucent table, lead apron and similar x-ray facilities should be available. There may well be safety regulations preventing the use of this piece of equipment in the outpatient department. However, it is essential that it is available in the operating theatre together with a lesion generator suitable for cordotomy, trigeminal radiofrequency coagulation, facetectomy, and a block aid monitor. Usually the lesion generator has stimulating facilities which can act as a block aid monitor. Additional special equipment such as needles of various lengths, pituitary injection needles, electrodes, electrical equipment of the transcutaneous neuromodulating type and an acupuncture electrical stimulator are also necessary.

Normal equipment would include a variety of needles, sterilizing fluids, anaesthetic solutions (including lignocaine in various strengths, 0·5, 1 and 2 per cent both plain and with adrenaline; bupivacaine (Marcain) 0·25 and 0·5 per cent plain and with adrenaline; 2 per cent benzocaine in oil; and 6 per cent Urethane) and disposable packs, trays, swabs, towels and the like. Solutions of phenol in iophendylate injection (Myodil) 1 in 20 and 1 in 15, phenol in glycerin 1 in 20 and 1 in 15, and solutions of phenol in water or saline, 2, 6 and 8 per cent will be necessary.

A number of facts are worth recording. All the successful pain clinics have been built on the effective treatment of inoperable cancer pain. If pain of this type is relieved then cases of other types of pain will automatically follow from the doctors concerned. It is also axiomatic that, in the early stages of a pain relief centre, only the most seriously ill patients (i.e. those most ill from inoperable cancer pain) will be sent and it is important not only to obtain good results but not to have these patients die as a result of treatment even though they are in poor condition. It is also important to call the clinic the pain *relief* clinic and in all the notices and stationery of the clinic the word 'relief' should be prominent.

The salient point of a pain clinic and the whole purpose of the exercise is for the patient in pain to meet the physician interested in relieving him of his pain. All else is secondary. The physician may not have a perfect knowledge of pain mechanisms or syndromes but this will correct itself with time. Bearing in mind the stage which this speciality of pain relief has reached, the over-riding consideration is for interested physicians to start clinics and to see patients, listen to their complaints and treat them by the simplest and most effective means available.

Further Reading

Bonica, J. J. and Black, R. G. (1974). The management of a pain clinic. In: *Relief of Intractable Pain*, pp. 116–129. Ed. by M. Swerdlow. Excerpta Medica, London and Amsterdam.
Churcher, M. D. (1973) Pain clinic cases. *Practitioner* **210**, 243.
McEwen, B. W., de Wilde, F. W., Dwyer, B., Woodforde, J. M., Bleasel, K. and Connelley, T. J. (1965) The pain clinic: a clinic for the management of intractable pain. *Medical Journal of Australia* **1**, 676.
Swerdlow, M. (1967). Four year's pain clinic experience. *Anaesthesia* **22**, 568.
Swerdlow, M. (1972). The pain clinic. *British Journal of Clinical Practice* **26**, 403.
Swerdlow, M., Mehta, M. D. and Lipton, S. (1978). Current views on the therapy of chronic pain. 'The role of the anaesthetist in chronic pain management'. *Anaesthesia* **33**, 250–257.

7

Measurement of pain

It is quite impossible to appreciate the degree of pain a particular patient is suffering. First of all, there are differences in appreciation of pain between patients. This was well understood many years ago by Keele (1962), who used his algometer (a plunger with an adjustable spring for increasing pressure upon the forehead) to determine pain perception and pain intolerance level. He found there was an average group of patients, a group of hypo-reactors who did not appreciate pain easily and a group of hyper-reactors who did appreciate pain easily. The latter group would naturally require larger doses and more powerful drugs to relieve their pain than the others. There is no method of picking out these patients before they have pain and a fine judgement must be maintained by the doctor who is treating non-malignant pain in deciding how much pain actually is present, what the patient's pain appreciation is, what strength of drug can reasonably be given, and what 'benefit', if any, is the patient getting out of the pain.

The 10 centimetre line

It is possible to decide how a patient's pain is varying on a day-to-day basis, or even from hour to hour, by the use of the 10 centimetre line (Fig. 7.1). This is literally a line of 10 cm length, with one end labelled no pain and the other end labelled the most severe pain that can be imagined. The patient is asked to make a mark along this line signifying the level of the pain he is experiencing at that moment. Although it is not possible to compare one patient with another using this method, it does provide a satisfactory and fairly accurate method of assessing pain in the same patient from time to time. There are a number of safeguards which must be borne in mind. The writing must be either at the end of the line or continuously under the line with the words 'no pain' and the words 'severe pain' running into each other. If the words are bunched up at either end then the patients will tend to make their marks where the writing ends or begins.

45

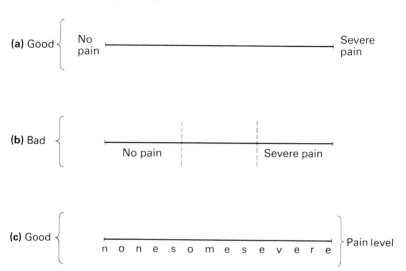

Fig. 7.1 10 centimetre lines. In (b) the patients tend to mark at the dotted lines

Some other methods

There are other methods of assessing pain and most suffer from the problem that, while they provide a reasonable measurement of the same person's pain, they do not allow comparison between patients. One method is to raise a blister on the skin and paint it with known concentrations of irritant solutions—potassium solutions are very effective; another is focusing a heat beam on to a black-painted portion of the skin, whilst stimulating the teeth with electric current (pulp stimulation) is a third method.

Tourniquet pain ratio

A useful method is to produce (experimentally) a pain in the patient and to ask him to match his normal pain against this standard. This is the technique developed by Smith, *et al.* (1968) called the 'submaximum effort tourniquet technique', and advocated by Sternbach (1974) as the 'tourniquet pain ratio'. In this test a blood pressure cuff is placed on the non-dominant arm and the blood is drained from it by a rubber bandage which is not removed until the cuff pressure is above systolic. The cuff is kept above systolic, and the patient squeezes a hand exerciser slowly twenty times, and then a stopwatch is started. The time taken for the patient to appreciate pain of an intensity equal to his normal pain is noted, and the test continues until the patient's pain reaches a level which cannot be tolerated further. The two levels of pain are known as the clinical pain level and the maximum tolerance level.

Sternbach reports on the excellent reliability of this method which, provided there is no alteration of treatment, has a reproducibility of the order of 0·8, which is statistically highly significant and confirms its reliability. Sternbach derives a tourniquet pain ratio score by dividing the clinical pain level time by the maximum tolerance time and multiplying by 100.

This method has advantages in that it provides the doctor with a method of estimating pain levels apart from word descriptions. For instance, to the patient who insists his pain is terribly severe but in whom the tourniquet pain ratio score shows the pain to be much less than he says, the physician can reply with truth that he does know how much pain he has and it's not too bad (Sternbach, 1974).

Further reading

Beecher, H. K. (1959). Measurement of Subjective Responses. Quantitative effects of drugs. Oxford University Press, New York and London.

Chapman, C. R. (1976). Measurement of pain: problems and issues. In: *Advances in Pain Research and Therapy*, Vol. 1, pp. 345–353. Ed. by J. J. Bonica and D. Albe-Fessard. Raven Press, New York.

Charpentier, J. (1968). Analysis and measurement of pain in animals. In: *Pain*, pp. 171–200. Ed. by A. Soulairac, J. Cahn and J. Charpentier. Academic Press, New York and London.

Cox, G. B. and Chapman, C. R. (1976). Multivariate analysis of pain data. In: *Advances in Pain Research and Therapy*, Vol. 1, pp. 363–373. Ed. by J. J. Bonica and D. Albe-Fessard. Raven Press, New York.

Keele, C. A. (1962). *The Assessment of Pain in Man and Animals*. Ed. by C. A. Keele and R. Smith. E. & S. Livingstone, Edinburgh.

Rollman, G. B. (1976). Signal detection theory assessment of pain modulation; a critique. In: *Advances in Pain Research and Therapy*, Vol. 1, pp. 355–362. Ed. by J. J. Bonica and D. Albe-Fessard. Raven Press, New York.

Smith, G. M., Lowenstein, E., Hubbard, J. H. and Beecher, H. K. (1968). Experimental pain produced by the submaximal effort tourniquet technique. Further evidence of validity. *Journal of Pharmacology and Experimental Therapeutics* **163**, 468–474.

Swets, J. A. (Ed.) (1964). *Signal Detection and Recognition by Human Observers*. John Wiley, New York.

Sternbach, R. A. (1974). Diagnostic procedures and predictions. In: *Pain Patients: traits and treatment*, p. 82. Academic Press, New York and London.

8

Pain in the head

Headache

Most headaches are self-limiting disturbances which arise in the muscles or blood vessels of the scalp or neck, and only a small number are due to structural changes. It is important to realize that the intensity of a headache is unrelated to the presence or absence of structural disease and it is the pattern of pain development which is the key to diagnosis.

There are only a few structures within the cranium which are sensitive to pain; these include the dura, the arteries and the veins, while the fifth, ninth and tenth cranial nerves will produce pain if they are directly involved in a disease process. Stimulation of any of the remaining cranial nerves and the brain itself does not produce pain. The dura and the vessels of the anterior and middle fossae and the upper surface of the tentorium are supplied through the fifth cranial nerve; pain from these structures is referred to the cranial distribution, which means that the pain is referred to the frontal and the retro-orbital regions. In similar fashion, the inferior surface of the tentorium, the dura and the vessels of the posterior fossa are supplied through the ninth and tenth cranial nerves and the upper two cervical nerves, so that pain from these structures is referred to the occipital and nuchal regions.

Pain in the head and neck can arise from any of the layers of the scalp and, in particular, from the muscles or blood vessels. Other structures include the nasal sinuses, the eye, the middle ear, the teeth, the cervical nerve roots, the cervical facet joints and the temporomandibular joints. Each of these tends to have its own type of pain and their principal characteristics are:

1. *The blood vessels.* Headaches arising from the blood vessels of the head and neck—either intracranial or extracranial—have a throbbing quality and the extent of the pain depends on the number of vessels involved.

2. *The muscles of the scalp* produce pain which is described as a tightness or a pressure.

3. *Sinus pain* is felt as an aching deep in the face around the orbit, forehead or maxilla, depending upon which sinuses are affected. The pain of infection is localized and does not remit whilst that of malignant disease is much more severe and diffuse.

48

4. *Trigeminal pain* and other types of neuralgias are characterized by severe lancinating pain. These jabs of pain are very fleeting and between them the patient is free from pain.

5. *Psychological pain*, often associated with depression, is usually a dull ache, lasting for hours or days without much variation.

Thus the history indicates the diagnosis.

Tension headache

Muscle contraction headache, or tension headache, is probably the commonest of all the types of headache seen. It is due to a persistent contraction of scalp muscles, occipital muscles or of the masseters, and it produces a pain usually described as a heavy weight pressing on the head, as a band of tightness round the head or as a dull ache. When fully developed, it is really severe and may become widespread. It is common in young women.

These symptoms are the result of fatigue, tension or stress, and the patients often recognize this and may treat themselves symptomatically. On examination, the patients appear to be tense and often have an inability to relax the limb muscles. This condition may occur as a result of the patient's occupation and it is prevalent in commercial travellers, lorry drivers and others who keep their head in one position for long periods of time.

The double insertion of the scalp muscles into the supraorbital region and into the occipital region means that these two areas become very tender from prolonged contraction of the muscles, and simple measures such as exercise, reduction of mental or physical tension, voluntarily relaxing muscles and simple analgesic drugs will usually relieve this type of pain. In some patients, the process is long standing, and they may have to make adjustments to their life-style.

Migraine

The treatment of true migraine proceeds in logical fashion, depending upon a clear understanding of the underlying pathological process (or as much of it as is known to date) so that the manner in which drugs are used is carefully thought out. Thus if speedy action of the vasoconstrictor, ergotamine, is needed, an inhaler is used; if a long slow action, a suppository. If a serotonin antagonist is to be used, then there is a selection available, and if these common methods fail there are other, less specific, drugs to use.

In a basic plan for treating patients in pain there must be a scheme of treatment; an escalating orderly process with the simple, safe methods tried first.

Migraine can be divided into classic and common migraine. In both types the headache is preceded or accompanied by transitory disturbances of cerebral function (prodromal symptoms), and it is these which distinguish it from other forms of vascular headache. The preceding symptoms are produced by spasm of cerebral blood vessels and the type produced depends on the area of brain or brain stem which these blood vessels supply. Frequently there are visual disturbances produced by spasm of a posterior cerebral artery with resultant ischaemia of an occipital pole, while if brain stem function is disturbed, as in basilar migraine, nausea is usually present associated with disturbed brain stem functions such as vertigo, autonomic disturbance, cranial nerve palsies and paraesthesiae.

If the middle cerebral artery is involved, then hemiplegic migraine results, shown by a slowly spreading sensory disturbance, sometimes associated with paresis beginning in one part of the body and spreading to other areas. The spread accurately follows the anatomic relationship of the cerebral tissue supplied by the middle cerebral artery so that this is the type of sensory disturbance which starts in an arm, spreads to the shoulder, thence to the face and lips and eventually to the leg.

Classic migraine will first produce premonitory symptoms and, as these are settling in perhaps one-half to one hour, the migrainous headache develops. This headache is produced by dilatation of the branches of the external carotid artery, including its dural and extracerebral blood vessels, and the site of pain is determined solely by the anatomy of the blood vessels involved. These headaches often start locally and spread more widely as additional blood vessels become involved. The characteristic pain of the migrainous headache is its throbbing character. It is only the larger vessels which dilate; the small cutaneous vessels remain contracted and the patient usually looks pale during an attack.

The arteries affected vary in successive migraine attacks; if they do not, then the patient should be investigated to make sure there is no intracranial pathology.

Common migraine does not necessarily show this classical pattern but the patient has attacks in which there may be no premonitory symptoms at all, attacks where cerebral symptoms follow the onset of the headache, or attacks where they run together.

Migraine headaches are due to an increased reactivity of cerebral blood vessels and this in turn is due to a sensitivity to circulating serotonin. This vasoconstrictor substance is normally contained in the platelets and at the beginning of an attack there is a slight increase of serum serotonin concentration. As the headache develops, the serotonin level falls (Curran, Hinterberger and Lance, 1965). The initial constriction of the cerebral blood vessels produces an ischaemia of the cerebral cortex and brain stem, with temporary diminution in function; this produces the aura in the classic migraine, while later the lowered level of serotonin produces the extracerebral blood vessel dilatation and the headache. Why only certain blood vessels should contract or dilate is not known.

Many of the drugs used in treatment are serotonin antagonists but most mild migraine headaches respond to simple analgesics; these are best used in combination with the traditional remedy, ergotamine tartrate 1–2 mg, which is usually given as a sublingual tablet. This drug has a vasoconstrictor action and relieves the headache dramatically in many cases. To be effective it should be taken early in an attack before the headache develops because, once the extracerebral vessels dilate, ergotamine is ineffective.

Some patients use an ergotamine inhaler which gives rapid absorption; the daily dose must not exceed 4 mg. Care must be taken with ergotamine given by other methods and, because of its vasoconstrictor effect on peripheral vessels, the drug must be avoided in patients who have Raynaud's disease, coronary arterial disease or are pregnant.

In patients who wake up with migraine or who require prophylactic ergotamine because of frequent severe attacks, ergotamine suppositories may be useful.

When the ergotamine drugs are not effective, then the serotonin antagonist methysergide (Deseril) 1–4 mg daily can be used. This is an excellent drug but it has definite disadvantages as it can produce retroperitoneal, pleural or cardiac fibrosis and so it must not be used continuously. It is quite safe if the dose does not exceed 4 mg daily and if it is given for not more than five months at a time. There should be a one month period when the drug is withdrawn. This greatly reduces the side effects.

Other serotonin antagonists are cyproheptadine (Periactin) 8–32 mg daily or pizotifen (Sanomigran) 1–3 mg daily. These drugs do not cause fibrosis but do stimulate the appetite and may increase weight for this reason.

Another prophylactic drug is clonidine (Dixarit) 0·025–0.075 mg daily. This drug increases the vasomotor stability of blood vessels by its central action but occasionally produces mild hypotensive symptoms.

There are two further comments to make on drug therapy in migraine. When all else has been tried in migraine without good relief, it is worth while trying propranolol (Inderal). This is an adrenergic β-blocking drug, which blocks the β-receptors and prevents any adrenaline dilatation of blood vessels. Further, monoamine oxidase inhibitors raise blood serotonin levels and also can be used to treat resistant cases (Anthony and Lance, 1969). When this drug is used, the patient's diet must be supervised carefully to avoid ingesting those amines with adrenergic-potentiating properties.

Migrainous neuralgia (cluster headache)

This condition, as in migraine, is due to a disordered reactivity of cranial blood vessels. The two syndromes are quite distinct both on clinical and biochemical grounds. In particular, in migrainous neuralgia the cerebral blood vessels are unaffected and there are no premonitory symptoms produced by vasospasm, such as flashing lights, and nausea, vomiting and gastrointestinal symptoms do not occur.

The pain of migrainous neuralgia affects the face, the forehead, or the orbital region, and is unilateral with no radiation. In any particular episode a single site is usually affected, although very occasionally the site of pain will change. It is most unusual for both sides to be affected at the same time. The pain of migrainous neuralgia is much more localized than that of migraine while the intensity is much worse, being equalled only by the severest of migraine headache. It is a most intense throbbing pain with cutaneous vasodilatation of the cheek; in addition, the conjunctival vessels may dilate, as may vessels of the nasal mucosa on the affected side, producing a nasal obstruction or a running nostril. The combination of a sore watering eye with a blocked nose is common.

This particular syndrome affects people of all ages from puberty upwards and, unlike migraine, males are more commonly affected than females.

There is a pattern of attack that is seen in almost all the sufferers. The patient is woken up at a constant time every night, often around 2:00 a.m. The attacks stop quite suddenly after a few weeks and the patient is then free from them for some time. In some patients the attacks start during the day and in others they are quite irregular.

The sympathetic nerve fibres to the pupil pass through the base of the skull around the internal carotid artery; when this vessel dilates, the nerves are compressed in the bony canal and it is not uncommon for a patient with migrainous neuralgia to have ipsilateral ptosis and a small pupil. This is a partial Horner's syndrome resulting from damage to the sympathetic nerve fibres. In some patients with long histories of migrainous neuralgia, there may be a permanent Horner's syndrome.

Serotonin levels remain unchanged during the headache of migrainous neuralgia (Anthony and Lance, 1971) but histamine levels are raised. Conversely, histamine levels do not change during migraine attacks while serotonin levels do. If histamine is injected in patients who suffer from migrainous neuralgia during an attack, then pain is precipitated; if it is injected during the remission period, headache is not usually produced. It thus appears that histamine is a precipitating factor when the blood vessels have been sensitized by some other means.

The treatment of migrainous neuralgia is to relieve the painful dilatation of the cranial arteries causing the pain, and the drugs used are the same as those in migraine. As with migraine, ergotamine tartrate should be given before the vessels are fully dilated but, as there are no premonitory symptoms with migrainous neuralgia, this is difficult. For this reason, ergotamine tartrate should be given by injection, or ergotamine can be given by inhalation (this route is just as rapid and probably is the better method of administration).

As might be expected, ergotamine suppositories are useful in the prevention of nocturnal attacks and in any case prophylactic therapy can be carried out during a bout of migrainous neuralgia. Dihydroergotamine 1–2 mg t.d.s. is used for this purpose but often methysergide (Deseril) is necessary and can be used in higher doses than for migraine up to 8–10 mg daily. This high dose of methysergide may be used for only a few weeks at the most.

Other causes of vascular headache

The majority of headaches are quite benign and this is commonly understood by the population at large. However, very rarely, headache is a symptom of a serious condition and this must be kept in mind when treating a patient with headache. Brief mention is now made of these other rare causes of headache but it is emphasized that tension headache, migraine, cluster headaches and trigeminal neuralgia account for the majority of pains in the head.

Vascular headaches

These can be produced by a number of conditions, of which malignant hypertension with papilloedema causes the most severe headache which has a throbbing character. A moderate rise in blood pressure will aggravate migraine but, normally, moderate hypertension does not cause headache.

Meningeal irritation

Due to either bacterial meningitis or a subarachnoid haemorrhage, meningeal irritation can be acute. This produces severe, constant headache felt in the occipital and nuchal areas, which becomes more generalized as the meningeal irritation spreads out from the posterior fossa. Often there is neck rigidity and a positive Kernig's sign.

Raised intracranial pressure

This is due to traction and displacement of blood vessels by the enlarging ventricular system. The more rapid the rise in pressure, the more likely is headache to occur. Any procedure which increases intracranial pressure exacerbates the headache so that stooping, coughing, sneezing, etc., make the condition worse. In the later stages the headache will be associated with vomiting, papilloedema and cranial nerve palsies. Any progressive symptoms of this type call for the urgent investigation of the patient.

Cerebral tumours

These usually produce symptoms when rapidly increasing in size. In those cases where the tumour (such as a meningioma) expands slowly, there is little in the way of symptoms until the tumour presses on vulnerable structures or suddenly increases in size.

Intracranial aneurysm

An intracranial aneurysm is a special form of cerebral tumour, and a rapid expansion of an intracranial aneurysm can produce severe, well localized, throbbing pain. Most aneurysms do not give any localizing signs before they rupture. The commonest site for an aneurysm is at the origin of the posterior communicating artery near the third cranial nerve. At this site an expanding aneurysm usually produces a third nerve palsy which can be almost diagnostic.

Subarachnoid haemorrhage

In subarachnoid haemorrhage there is severe headache and the diagnosis not usually in doubt.

Subdural haematoma

This can extend over a large area of the cerebral hemisphere and, as it may cause widespread irritation of the meninges, it is often associated with headache. The pain is at the site of the lesion and a subdural haematoma should be suspected in any patient with a persistent unilateral headache who has a progressive or fluctuating history of drowsiness or intellectual alteration. A subdural haematoma is often preceded by a head injury but the patient and his relatives may not remember or be aware of this.

Temporal arteritis

As already mentioned, most headaches are of no great clinical significance, but there is one which is of particular importance: temporal arteritis.

Temporal arteritis is often associated with polymyalgia rheumatica, the salient features of which are that it occurs in elderly or middle-aged patients and is more common in women. The muscles of the body and proximal limbs are affected and morning stiffness is usually severe, there is fatigue, depression and loss of weight.

The danger in polymyalgia rheumatica is that a temporal arteritis may develop, shown by scalp tenderness and eventually generalized headache with loss of pulsation of the temporal artery. The erythrocyte sedimentation rate (ESR) is greatly raised but if the condition is suspected it should be treated before the ESR result is known, because there is a great danger of sudden and irreversible blindness due to an arteritis involving the ophthalmic arteries. The treatment is by large doses of corticosteroids, such as prednisone up to 60 mg daily, depending upon the effect on the ESR.

Other conditions

Headaches are also produced from diseases of the sinuses, the temporomandibular joint, Paget's disease of bone, and from the cervical vertebrae.

It is obvious that every headache cannot be studied in detail but a full physical examination should be carried out and those patients who have long-standing headache, unilateral headache, fits, or physical signs should be investigated.

Trigeminal neuralgia

Classically, trigeminal neuralgia is known as tic douloureux because, during a severe paroxysm of pain, the face becomes contorted in agony. The classic trigeminal neuralgia is a condition diagnosed relatively easily, as certain clinical features are commonly present.

It is rarely seen before the age of 40 and two-thirds of the patients are aged over 50. It occurs more frequently in women than in men, with a ratio of about 2:1. The pain is of great severity, occurring in bouts which may last from a few days to a few months. During an attack there is a succession of paroxysmal pains confined to one, two or all of the trigeminal nerve divisions on one side of the face. The pain does not cross the midline and trigger points are often present. Touching, speaking, chewing or swallowing may initiate a paroxysm.

The attacks are always brief, lasting only a few minutes, and after a paroxysm there may be a dull ache in the face, which disappears fairly rapidly. Between paroxysms there is no pain; some patients describe a persistent dull ache after they have had an attack, but in the classic condition this is not so.

Often the pain is confined to one division so that a pain starting in the cheek, shooting towards the upper jaw, lip and under the eye, denotes a second division trigeminal neuralgia whilst third division neuralgia starts anterior to the ear and shoots down to the cheek and tongue. There is no fixed direction of this shooting pain; it can start in the chin or tongue and shoot towards the ear. First division pain is rare on its own but may be present combined with pain in one of the other areas.

The symptoms can remit spontaneously and the patient may continue many years without further neuralgia. Usually, the interval between attacks gets shorter as time goes on and eventually the patient demands treatment. Occasionally, young people below the age of 40 are affected; in such a case an organic disease should be suspected, such as multiple sclerosis.

Between the attacks of trigeminal neuralgia no abnormal physical signs will be found. If there is any alteration of sensation in the distribution of the trigeminal nerve, then an intracranial lesion must be suspected.

Treatment

Drug therapy

Carbamazepine (Tegretol) has simplified the treatment of trigeminal neuralgia. This drug has a membrane threshold stabilizing effect on the spinal trigeminal nucleus and is believed to reduce synaptic transmission as a result. It is related to the tricyclic antidepressants of the imipramine type and has toxic effects which include hypomanic excitement, extrapyramidal symptoms, peripheral atropine-like reactions and, occasionally, orthostatic hypotension. It is to be used with great care in patients who have glaucoma and should not be used in combination with a monoamine oxidase inhibitor (Williams, 1977).

In particular, blood dyscrasias may occur with this drug, including agranulocytosis and aplastic anaemia. Great difficulties arise in treating patients if any of these dyscrasias occur, especially when it causes a reduction of the platelets. Under these circumstances neither injection nor operation can be carried out to relieve the pain; replacement blood therapy must be instituted before operation.

The rationale for the method of using carbamazepine (Tegretol) is not generally understood. It should be given continuously until pain is relieved and continued for several weeks after the patient has been free from pain, when it can be reduced slowly. Normally the patient requires 600 mg daily in divided doses, but some patients will require nearly twice this dosage. High doses (over 600 mg) can be expected to produce drowsiness and ataxia, and elderly patients and their relatives must be warned about this. Usually the ataxic complications become less pronounced after a few days. The usual mistake made is that the patient does not take the drug prophylactically; if it is taken only during a paroxysm of pain it will be valueless.

Alternatives to carbamazepine are phenytoin (Epanutin) in equivalent dose, or, when there is a partial response to carbamazepine, then clonazepam (Rivotril) is worth trying in small doses (0·5 mg t.d.s.). All these drugs are used as anti-epileptics, which suggests that the condition is due to a discharge in centrally located trigeminal neurones (King, 1967), but some authorities believe the aetiology of the condition is peripheral (Kerr, 1967).

All patients on carbamazepine therapy should have weekly red blood cell counts, white cell counts and platelet counts for four weeks. After this period it can be carried out regularly at four- to five-weekly intervals. Despite this regime there will be an occasional patient who develops a fulminating leucopenia but usually there will be some warning that the white cells are being reduced.

Surgical treatment

When medical treatment has failed, or when medical treatment has been continued for a long period with carbamazepine or it is thought to be dangerous because of the risk of blood dyscrasias, surgical treatment can be tried. The trigeminal nerve and its pathways can be sectioned in a number of places—at the periphery, at the main branches and at the root. It must be emphasized that any of these procedures will produce anaesthesia in the part of the face served by the particular portion of the nerve sectioned. In some patients this numbness is distressing and, if the trigeminal neuralgia is not too severe or too frequent, they often prefer the pain to the numbness. A diagnostic block with local anaesthetic will often give the patient some idea of the loss of sensation they will have from a permanent procedure.

Peripheral nerves are usually injected at the infraorbital foramen or at the supraorbital notch. More usually, mandibular or maxillary nerve block can be performed at a number of sites—described later. After diagnostic blocks, these nerves are destroyed with a neurolytic agent such as alcohol or phenol. The trigeminal ganglion can be approached through the foramen ovale and injections made into or close to the ganglion.

All these peripheral procedures, whether there is neurolytic destruction of the nerve or surgical section of it, suffer from the defect that regeneration of nerve takes place and the pain will recur.

The gasserian ganglion is invaginated into a double fold of dura; if the needle is advanced until cerebrospinal fluid is obtained, then selective blocking of one or other division of the trigeminal nerve can be obtained by positioning the patient and using hypobaric alcohol (Penman, 1953), hyperbaric phenol in glycerine, or phenol in wax solutions (Jefferson, 1963). In the surgical method the nerve is sectioned proximal to the ganglion so that regeneration of the nerve does not occur and thus pain cannot return.

Radiofrequency coagulation

The most modern method of treatment of trigeminal neuralgia avoids surgery but obtains the same benefit as the root section. A new technique, called radiofrequency coagulation of the trigeminal nerve roots, is performed with a needle electrode which is passed through the foramen ovale from a point 3–4 cm lateral to the corner of the mouth and inserted until cerebrospinal fluid is obtained. The needle is insulated except for the terminal 5 mm. X-ray control is used and the needle electrode tip is placed amongst the trigeminal rootlets (Fig. 8.1). Stimulation at about 50 Hz will be felt by the patient

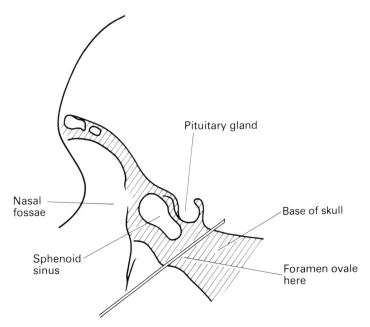

Fig. 8.1   Needle electrode position for thermocoagulation of trigeminal rootlets.

as a tingling or pain in some portion of the face and the needle can be adjusted until this sensation occurs in the painful area. Radiofrequency heat coagulation is then carried out, testing between each coagulation for developing analgesia (see p. 118).

With this technique, analgesia can be obtained without removing all sensation in the face and the patient can be left with dense analgesia rather than anesthesia.

The procedure is carried out under 'anaesthetic sleep' and is rather lengthy because the patient sleeps during the painful parts of the procedure and must wake up to give rational answers when the stimulation testing is being performed. Time must be allowed for proper recovery between each 'sleep'.

One of the great problems following destruction of the trigeminal pathways is the condition known as anaesthesia dolorosa. In this the patient has a completely anaesthetized face, or portion of face, and yet has pain in that area. Using the differential radiofrequency coagulation of the trigeminal roots a little sensation is left and it is claimed that this prevents the development of anaesthesia dolorosa (Sweet and Wepsic, 1974).

Glossopharyngeal neuralgia

This is a rare condition corresponding to trigeminal neuralgia. The paroxysms of pain in this condition are precipitated by swallowing and by tongue movements. It can be treated by glossopharyngeal nerve block or by surgical section of the nerve.

References

Anthony, M. and Lance, J. W. (1969). Monoamine oxidase inhibition in the treatment of migraine. *Archives of Neurology* **21**, 263.
Anthony, M. and Lance, J. W. (1971). Histamine and serotonin in cluster headache. *Archives of Neurology* **25**, 225.
Curran, D. A., Hinterberger, H. and Lance, J. W. (1965). Total plasma serotonin, 5-hydroxyindole acetic acid and *p*-hydroxy-*m*-methoxymandelic acid excretion in normal and migrainous subjects. *Brain* **88**, 997.
Jefferson, A. (1963). Trigeminal root and ganglion injections using phenol in glycerine for the relief of trigeminal neuralgia. *Journal of Neurology, Neurosurgery and Psychiatry* **26**, 345.
Kerr, F. W. (1967). Evidence for a peripheral etiology of trigeminal neuralgia. *Journal of Neurosurgery* **26**, 168.
King, R. B. (1967). Evidence for a central etiology of tic douloureux. *Journal of Neurosurgery* **26**, 175.
Penman, J. (1953). Some developments in the technique of trigeminal injection. *Lancet*, **i**, 760.
Sweet, W. H. and Wepsic, J. G. (1974). Controlled thermocoagulation of the trigeminal ganglion and rootlets for differential destruction of pain fibres. *Journal of Neurosurgery* **40, 143.**
Williams, N. E. (1977). The role of drug therapy. In: *Persistent Pain*, Vol. 1, p. 247. Ed. by S. Lipton. Academic Press, London and New York.

Further reading

Diamonds, S. and Dalessio, D. J. (1973). *The Practising Physician's approach to Headache*. Medcom Press, New York.
Lance, J. W. (1973). *The Mechanism and Management of Headache*. 2nd edn. Butterworths, London.

9
Rheumatic conditions

It has been estimated that in Britain only about 1 person in 50 will avoid rheumatic complaints by the age of 70. One might expect that tremendous efforts would be made to solve the problems posed by these diseases but such is not the case. Certainly the subject is not as neglected as previously but the money spent bears no relation to the cost in human suffering or to the actual financial loss of the sufferer and the nation.

An idea commonly accepted is that rheumatism is a British disease and is something which has to be accepted because it is incurable. However, there is much that can be done to relieve the resulting pain and disability.

It is not easy to provide relief, as in many cases the cause of the disease is unknown and the major symptom, pain, is always difficult to assess. When this is combined with frequent fluctuations in the severity of the particular rheumatic condition suffered, treatment becomes especially difficult. However, if one considers which areas of the body are affected by the rheumatic disease, it can be seen that the mechanical and moving parts are the ones involved. This means the bones, muscles, tendons and ligaments and their nervous and vascular connections. It also means that rest, support and even splinting will play a large part in treatment.

It is not my intention to work through a classification of the rheumatic diseases but it is important to pick out certain conditions in which pain is a major symptom.

Fibrositis

Fibrositis is the most common of rheumatic conditions and is usually classified as non-articular rheumatism or myofascial disease. There is pain and stiffness, especially in the large muscles, which are aggravated by immobility, fatigue, depression, cold and damp.

The pain is of an aching, diffuse type but localized situations, called trigger points, are often present where marked tenderness and pain are felt. The pain may be felt at a distance from the trigger point producing it, when it is known as referred pain (Kellgren, 1949). However, in many cases, pain is present in superficial bony places where ligaments or tendons are attached to bone. These places are called the enthesis. Conditions such as tennis elbow (Lawrence, 1977) and periarthritis of the shoulder come into this category.

The normal management of fibrositis is somewhat vague but what treatment there is includes rest, warmth, physiotherapy and drugs. The drugs used should be kept simple, utilizing analgesics and anti-inflammatory agents such as paracetamol, aspirin or proprionic derivatives such as naproxen. The more powerful anti-inflammatory drugs (e.g. indomethacin) should not be used early owing to their possible dangerous side effects. Injection of local anaesthetic solutions sometimes combined with steroids is often made into painful entheses or trigger points.

There are very interesting features of correspondence between the trigger points of the myofascial diseases and acupuncture points, and this merits some consideration.

Trigger points can be stimulated in various ways—by dry needling, by injecting hypertonic saline, by pressure, or by electrical stimulation. They are treated (or, rather, the pain they produce on stimulation can be treated) by injection of a local anaesthetic into the trigger point; often, once the pain has been relieved, it may not return for some time, long after the effect of the local anaesthetic has worn off. In some cases it does not return at all.

Strangely enough, the stimulation of acupuncture will also produce relief of pain; it is not difficult to see why, when a trigger point in the trapezius muscle close to the scapula is stimulated by dry needling and the referred pain in the side of the neck disappears, that the similarity with acupuncture is readily perceived (Melzack, 1975).

Travel and Rinzler (1952) and other workers in this field have recorded a large number of trigger points related to the patterns of pain in the myofascial conditions. There seem to be several features in common in that there are definite patterns of pain and trigger points in some conditions—so much so, that many patients without disease also have tenderness and even pain on pressing these points. Trigger points are not only related to painful superficial structures near to them but may be far away from the area in which they produce pain. They can be related to visceral pain, and the pain produced by pressure on any trigger point can last a very long time. Persistence of the stimulating effect is a common feature of trigger points.

In 1977, Melzack, Stilwell and Fox suggested that these features of trigger points resemble those of acupuncture points used for the relief of pain. They attempted to determine the correlation between trigger points and acupuncture points for pain, using the two criteria of their spatial distribution and the associated pain pattern. 'A remarkably high degree (71 per cent) of correspondence was found', and they considered that the two types of points were discovered independently and labelled differently, but were the same phenomenon. This is not a new concept; many doctors treating this type of pain have noted this correspondence but Melzack and his colleagues showed the numerical coincidence. They also suggest possible methods by which summating nervous mechanisms produce these effects.

They point out that transmission cells in the dorsal horn normally have a very wide receptive field but respond to a much smaller receptive field in normal activity. The input from the wider receptive field is usually inhibited but if it is not it triggers the transmission cell. A second method may be due to facilitation of local nerve transmission by activity in distant areas, and finally the intense stimulation produced by needling a trigger or acupuncture point may produce descending inhibition.

Further work remains to be done before this concept can be accepted but the scheme has great plausibility and is of practical use. (Acupuncture is discussed in Chapter 12.)

Soft tissue rheumatism

Soft tissue rheumatism is a conglomeration of many different conditions, some of which can be separated out into syndromes but all of which tend to merge one with another and to be somewhat imprecise.

Polymyalgia rheumatica is an example of the complex, diffuse presenting symptoms often found in these diseases. The clinical picture in this condition is well known but diagnosis is often delayed because there are few physical signs and no specific text. It occurs in middle-aged or elderly patients, more commonly in women than men, and its onset is acute, with pain and stiffness involving proximal muscles. Neck and shoulder are usually first, followed by the pelvic girdle muscles. Morning stiffness can be severe and there is constitutional upset. The development of temporal headache and scalp tenderness suggests giant cell arteritis, and tenderness, thickening and reduced pulsation in the superficial temporal arteries are very suggestive. A biopsy of this artery and an ESR will be diagnostic. Treatment should start immediately with large doses of steroids because delay may mean arteritis involving the ophthalmic artery and its branches, and irreversible blindness. However, the vasculitis is not confined to this artery and any artery may be affected, including intracerebral ones, producing hemiplegia.

This syndrome (if it can be called a syndrome) is imprecise, as polymyalgia rheumatica can merge, at a later stage, into a condition indistinguishable from rheumatoid arthritis. The question is then asked, are some cases of polymyalgia rheumatica a prodromal phase of, or a variant of, rheumatoid arthritis?

This vagueness of diagnosis tends to be present throughout the rheumatic conditions; nevertheless, some of these conditions are definite and the important painful ones are mentioned below, not so much to describe them but to point out the causal mechanisms and indicate the lines of treatment.

Tennis elbow

Tennis elbow is a commonly occurring condition due to inflammation or damage at the common tendinous origin of the extensor muscles of the wrist at the lateral epicondyle of the humerus. It is a good example of pain produced by inflammation at an enthesis.

Normally, the condition develops following trauma and, as might be expected, there is a corresponding injury to the common flexor tendon origin at the medial epicondyle of the humerus which is the 'golfers elbow'. The best test for the tennis elbow (apart from pressure at the enthesis) is to pronate the wrist with the hand closed and in ulnar deviation, and then extend the elbow. Pain will appear at the elbow when the test is positive. It is important to remember that, as the elbow joint is not involved, the elbow moves fully without pain.

Treatment of this condition corresponds to that in other types of rheumatic conditions in that rest of the affected part will usually cure the condition, at least if it is tried during the first attack; however, most patients will not, or cannot, afford this and opt for injection of steroids. Injection of an enthesis can be very painful and it is a kindness to add a little local anaesthetic to the solution.

Treatment by injection does not always cure the condition and as patients tend to become active too quickly, there is a relapse or recurrence and the condition becomes chronic.

The painful shoulder

There are three articulations involved in movement of the shoulder: the glenohumeral, the acromioclavicular and the clavicular. In addition, there is the gliding motion of the scapula over the thoracic cage. There are many structures around these joints, which include muscles, tendons and the sub-bursa. These structures, with the joint capsule and ligaments, form the rotator cuff which is a protective musculotendinous cuff. This cuff is prone to damage and the commonest lesion is a supraspinatus tendinitis but there are other associated lesions which include subacromial bursitis, adhesive capsulitis, bicipital tenosynovitis, degenerative conditions and direct injuries. The presenting symptoms are always pain and limited movement of the shoulder due to damage to these periarticular structures.

When severe, the periarthritic pain comes on rapidly and is severe and constant, often interfering with sleep as it is impossible for the patient to sleep on the affected side. In some varieties of periarthritis of the shoulder such as supraspinatus tendinitis the painful arc sign is positive. This means that there is pain on abduction of the arm on the shoulder in that part of the movement where the inflamed supraspinatus tendon moves under the acromion. Thus, part of the movement is free from pain and part of it is extremely painful. Symptomatic treatment is used and rest is important in the early stages. The arm is placed in a sling and analgesic drugs are used to cover the pain. The subacromial bursa or the affected tendon can be injected with local anaesthetic combined with a steroid. Sometimes the supraspinatus or biceps tendon ruptures, and while surgical repair can be made, the remaining disability may not be great enough to justify an operation.

A frozen shoulder or an adhesive capsulitis sometimes follows a coronary thrombosis or minor injury to the shoulder but it can occur without any previous damage. This is one of the reflex neurovascular dystrophies and fortunately tends to be a self-limiting condition. Repeated sympathetic blocks may help.

Crystal deposition arthropathy

Gout

Probably the most commonly known rheumatic condition, and certainly the most painful, is gout. This is the best known of the crystal deposition arthropathies but it is not the only one. In gout there is deposition of urate crystals but other types of crystals can be deposited in the tissues; these are calcium pyrophosphate dihydrate and hydroxyapatite. Urate and pyrophosphates can attack any joint but the hydroxyapatite crystals usually only involve the shoulder joint.

The clinical picture of gout is well known. Usually the patient is a male and he is woken from sleep by severe pain in the big toe, which is the site of the first attack in over 70 per cent of cases.

A typical acute attack lasts for one to two weeks and then resolves spontaneously. The pain is dull or burning, arising inside the joint, and it increases in severity over a few hours. In superficial joints, acute inflammatory signs are seen. The patient may not have another attack for weeks, months and sometimes years after the initial episode.

Gout is due to a mixture of genetic and environmental factors, and the principal feature is hyperuricaemia. Monosodium urate, which is produced in the body during purine catabolism, is a relatively insoluble compound and in gout there is over-production of this substance with defective excretion. If a metabolic abnormality is present, it is an inherited trait and the condition is a primary gout; other types, called secondary gout, are produced by causes such as increased cell catabolism.

In the acute attack, treatment must be immediate, the patient being put to bed or nursed in a chair with the affected joint immobilized and protected from pressure. A uric acid blood sample should be taken before drug treatment begins. Pain is dealt with by phenylbutazone 200 mg four times a day, or naproxen 750 mg initially followed by 250 mg six-hourly. These large doses are used to control the severe pain; they are then gradually reduced.

Long-term management involves using uricosuric drugs which increase urate excretion in combination with an inhibitor of uric acid production. Uricosuric drugs are probenecid 0·5–1·0 g twice a day, or sulphinpyrazone 400 mg daily. The dosage is determined individually by means of serial blood uric acid estimations. The purpose of treatment is to maintain a normal level of uric acid. In addition, as the enzyme xanthine oxidase is concerned with the oxidation of xanthine and hypoxanthine to uric acid and allopurinol is an inhibitor of the enzyme, this drug is given to inhibit uric acid production, the dose being 300 mg daily.

Pyrophosphate arthropathy

This occurs in sporadic form or in association with other diseases, such as hyperparathyroidism or diabetes mellitus. As in gout, there is an inherited trait which can resemble gout because it produces recurrent attacks of acute arthritis. However, these tend to affect the larger joints, especially the knees.

Pyrophosphate crystals form in the joint cartilage and eventually enter the synovial fluid and become coated with IgG globulin. This causes phagocytosis by polymorphonuclear leucocytes which migrate into the joint cavity. The leucocytes become damaged and release some of their lysosomal structure into the synovial cavity, which leads to a series of reactions producing an inflammation. Finally, an acute arthritis results which can be due either to gout or to pyrophosphate crystals.

Hydroxyapite crystal deposition

In hydroxyapatite crystal deposition, crystalline deposits form in the periarticular structures of bursae and tendons; the shoulder is a common site but it can occur around the hip, knee and finger joints. Apatite crystals have been found in the synovial fluid and presumably the course of events is similar to that of pyrophosphate arthropathy.

Rheumatoid arthritis

This condition, one of inflammatory polyarthritis, is more common in women than men but it is a common disease with a universal distribution and can develop at any age. There is a juvenile form of rheumatoid arthritis and, though the peak incidence is in middle life, it can occur for the first time in old age. It is a chronic erosive polyarthritis which affects symmetrical peripheral joints and tends to spread centripetally. Abnormal antibodies are often found in the blood and subcutaneous nodules occur around joints.

It is a systemic disease which affects all tissues and is accompanied by pyrexia, loss of weight, loss of appetite and depression. The synovial joints are usually the ones affected but the inflammatory reaction can occur in all connective tissues. Its aetiology is unknown and no cure is available. Treatment is designed to reduce the symptoms of the disease and to slow its progress. There are periods of exacerbation and remission, whilst the onset is insidious.

The principal symptoms are pain, stiffness, fatigue and often depression. In about 80 per cent of adult patients there are antibodies, called rheumatoid factors, present in the blood but these are not confined to rheumatoid arthritis, as similar antibodies occur in other diseases with no relationship to rheumatoid disease. There are tests for antibodies such as the latex fixation and sheep cell agglutination tests. Their main value is in prognosis and in distinguishing rheumatoid arthritis from the arthropathies of psoriasis and Reiter's disease, as neither of these conditions shows the rheumatoid factor. High titres of rheumatoid factors associated with subcutaneous nodule formation early in the disease indicate an unfavourable prognosis. Rheumatoid disease is an autoimmune disease but what factor is responsible for triggering off the autoimmune reaction is unknown.

In early cases the diagnosis can be difficult, some of the commoner diseases in the differential diagnosis being gout, acute rheumatism, systemic lupus erythematosus, polymyalgia rheumatica, septic arthritis, generalized osteoarthrosis, enteropathic arthropathy and Reiter's disease. It must be emphasized that this list is not meant to be comprehensive.

Those patients with acute polyarthritis require rest in bed and immobilization of inflamed joints. Anti-inflammatory drugs and analgesics will be supported by gold, penicillamine or chloroquine. Corticosteroids and immunosuppressants are used late in the disease.

Aspiration and injection of affected joints can be made and, after the acute inflammatory stage has settled, mobilization is started. Pain and stiffness are symptoms reducing mobility, while morning stiffness in particular, is a most troublesome condition. Aspirin is used for background therapy as it is both analgesic and anti-inflammatory but if the patient shows intolerance it must be withdrawn and paracetemol or a proprionic acid drug can be used. Indomethacin is especially useful at night, either orally or as a suppository to relieve nocturnal pain and morning stiffness, but it may produce gastric intolerance while phenylbutazone, an alternative, can produce blood dyscrasia.

As rheumatoid disease progresses, cumulative joint damage ensues, and this is shown by pain, deformity and impairment of function. Prophylactic surgery such as decompression synovectomy of a joint or tendon sheath can be carried out, while reconstructive surgery includes arthroplasty, osteotomy or arthrodesis.

Seronegative polyarthritis

Seronegative polyarthritis is the name given to a group of inflammatory joint diseases which are separate from rheumatoid disease. They include ankylosing spondylitis, psoriatic arthritis, Reiter's disease, ulcerative colitis arthritis, Behçet's syndrome and a number of others which have no rheumatoid factor in the blood. There is a familial relationship and certain features are common, including skeletal involvement, peripheral polyarthritis, ulceration of mucosal surfaces, inflammatory eye lesions and spinal ligament calcification.

The histocompatibility antigen, known as the HLA antigen, shows that there is a relationship between these conditions, the majority of which have an association with the HLA–B27 antigen. This is particularly so in the case of ankylosing spondylitis where the test for rheumatoid factor is negative but 96 per cent of cases are positive for the HLA–B27 antigen. There is a 7 per cent incidence of HLA–B27 antigen positive in the general population (Brewerton, 1975).

Ankylosing spondylitis

The best known of the seronegative polyarthritides group is ankylosing spondylitis, which affects young males between 16 and 40 years of age. Women can be affected. The patient has low back pain and a morning stiffness from immobility stiffness, while sciatica is present and alternates from leg to leg.

Pain around the thorax associated with reduced chest expansion is helpful diagnostically, and the normal lumbar curve is lost with spinal movements restricted in all directions. Recurrent iritis occurs in about 20 per cent of cases.

X-ray examination shows bilateral sacroiliitis in early cases; as the disease progresses, ligamentous calcification and ossification appear, spreading up the spine. This produces a typical appearance known as a bamboo spine. Complications include aortitis and apical pulmonary fibrosis. The ESR is raised in the active disease but when the disease is confined to the sacroiliac joints the ESR may be normal.

The treatment of ankylosing spondylitis is by the encouragement of activity which is carried out to maintain spinal mobility, and therefore physiotherapy, exercise, correct posture and daily breathing exercises are all important. Any pain and stiffness are relieved by indomethacin, naproxen of phenylbutazone. It is only when pain is not controlled by these measures that x-ray therapy is used.

Osteoarthrosis

Osteoarthrosis is the most common form of rheumatic degenerative joint disease, being universally present in the older age groups. One of the problems with this disease is that radiologically it can appear quite severe but as far as any clinical evidence is concerned it may be silent. The reason why a silent degenerative joint develops into a painful grating joint is unknown.

The common sites of involvement are the distal interphalangeal joints of the fingers, the proximal interphalangeal joints, the thumb carpometacarpal joints, the great toe metatarsophalangeal joints, the hips, knees, lumbar spine and cervical spine.

There are no specific investigations which are of value apart from radiological examination. The lesion starts in the articular cartilage which begins to break down due to separation, rupture and disorientation of collagen fibrils. Although progress of the lesion continues, simultaneous processes of repair and destruction proceed in the joints and as the disease progresses, cartilage gradually becomes eroded with possibly pyrophosphate and hydroxyapatite crystals being liberated into the joint.

The inflammatory reaction does not compare with that in acute gout or acute rheumatoid disease, being on a slower time scale, but as deterioration continues, the joint becomes unstable and there is ligamentous strain with the involved joints becoming swollen, having limited movement and being noisy and painful. The patient soon realizes that movement helps to relieve symptoms and that, for instance, nocturnal pain and stiffness can be relieved by getting up and moving about.

Osteoarthrosis is the final result of a multifactorial disease in which the ageing of tissues and stress or mechanical factors play a part. The treatment is purely symptomatic and, apart from protecting the affected joints from further damage, similar drug therapy as previously mentioned for rheumatoid disease is used. However, surgery has an important part to play in the treatment of certain joints, and the damaged hip joint in particular can be replaced by a prosthesis.

Back pain

There are an enormous number of causes for back pain. Benn and Wood (1975) state that in the United Kingdom over 13 million days were lost in the period from 1969 to 1970, because of back pain, accounting for 43 per cent of instances of absence from work due to rheumatic conditions.

Back pain is related to spinal movements and posture, and is relieved by rest. Coughing, sneezing and defaecation tend to increase the pain. Thus if pain is due to mechanical factors then it is increased during activity and decreased during rest, while conditions such as ankylosing spondylitis have an opposite effect where movement decreases pain and rest increases it. (In the case of ankylosing spondylitis, in addition there will be an increase in immobility stiffness.)

A full history is taken and this may suggest the diagnosis. A complete physical examination must be made, which means that the patient must remove all his clothes so that the spinal column can be properly examined. In this way posture and movements and whether these are stiff or painful can be seen easily. Particular points to note are: does the pelvis tilt, is the normal lumbar curve flattened, is a scoliosis present, is percussion of the spinous processes painful and is there any local deformity visible. The spinal movements are carefully observed and it is noted that often they are not restricted in all directions; for instance, in a prolapsed lumbar intervertebral disc, forward flexion is usually painful although the patient can carry out extension and rotation without great difficulty and the straight leg raising test (Lasègue's test) is usually positive.

If the patient can flex fairly normally but extension is painful, then it is most unlikely that a prolapsed lumbar intervertebral disc is present but rather that the pain arises at the zygoapophyseal joints (the facet joints).

In the cervical spine there are similar abnormalities of movement and, again, except for ankylosing spondylitis and severe spondylosis, these are not always restricted in all directions. If pain is severe in the neck and is due to structural disease, a well fitting cervical collar can be used. This will support the head on the neck, limit movement and reduce pain but it is most important that psychoneurotic patients should not be put into a cervical collar or a lumbar support. This type of patient can usually be distinguished by his general reactions during the taking of the history and the physical examination; conversely, a patient with organic pain must not be treated as a psychoneurotic patient.

One of the problems with the use of a cervical collar is that, even when worn by a patient with no cervical disease at all, after some time the patient feels insecure without it. The head is a heavy weight which is not quite balanced on a thin bony column and it is kept in equilibrium by the action of muscles. Using a collar relieves the muscles of constant work and after being worn for some time the patient may feel the head is unstable without it.

Laboratory tests depend on the history and the results of the examination but special tests should include a full blood count, ESR, serum acid and alkaline phosphatases, and examination of the urine. Radiology will include anteroposterior, lateral and oblique views of the affected spine; wider views may be useful, so the sacroiliac joints, the hip joints or the entire pelvis, including the lumbosacral region, may be x-rayed. In the cervical region, flexion and extension x-rays are sometimes useful to demonstrate movement or subluxation. The normal anteroposterior diameter of the vertebral foramen is 15 mm or more and this measurement may vary with posture.

Specialized radiological methods use contrast media which outline the spinal cord and spinal nerves. There are two types of these, oily solutions such as iophendylate (Myodil) and metrizamide which is water-soluble. The benefits of the water soluble radio-opaque dye is that being water soluble it is readily absorbed in about five hours. The oily solution remains *in situ* unless deliberately removed. Although iophendylate does gradually resorb it can produce an arachnoiditis in some patients.

An injection of radio-opaque material can be made into the substance of an intervertebral disc, this radiological method being known as discography and will show tears in or retropulsion of the disc.

Treatment

The treatment of back pain is similar to those of the peripheral joints and includes rest, supports, physiotherapy and analgesic and anti-inflammatory drugs. At a later stage surgery may be used, depending on the condition present. In the acute phase immediate rest is important. This should be on a firm bed and if it is not stiff enough fracture boards can be placed under the mattress to render the whole bed much firmer.

The treatment of back pain has largely become the treatment of the retropulsed vertebral disc in both cervical and lumbar regions. Dorsal discs occur only rarely so back pain at thoracic level is not usually ascribed to this cause.

Recently, attention has been focussed on other structures which might produce back pain and the most likely bony structure to do this is the posterior intervertebral joint (the facet or zygoapophyseal joint). This has a nerve supply from approximately the same level as the corresponding disc and is therefore likely to produce referred pain corresponding to the back pain but not to the root pain of retropulsed discs. It is a very vulnerable structure. To some extent, damage to the two structures can be distinguished relatively easily as patients with a retropulsed disc can usually extend their spine but not flex it, while patients with facet joint disease can usually flex their spine but not extend it; both can flex laterally. This does not imply that patients with either of these two complaints will be completely free from pain during either of these movements but, if taken slowly, even those in severe pain can demonstrate that bending one way is possible while the other is not.

Affections of the discs are regarded as rheumatic conditions; however, it is not just the intevertebral disc which is affected as the rheumatic process leading to a retropulsion of a disc is only part of a wider process (spondylosis deformans) which involves all the bony structures around the spinal canal.

Naturally this will include the facet joint which is immediately affected when a disc loses its incompressibility and movement occurs between the two vertebrae on either side of the disc. This movement is reflected in increased movement and strain of the facet joint. Thus often at one and the same level there is pathology present both in the disc and in the facet joint and one or other may predominate, or both may be at fault. In the latter case, if an abnormal retropulsed disc is removed surgically the root pain due to this may disappear but back pain may remain and this may be due to the facet joint. The treatment of pain from this cause is discussed in Chapter 16.

The intervertebral disc

An intervertebral disc consists of a cartilaginous plate, the nucleus pulposus and the annulus fibrosus. The cartilage plates merge into the cancellous bone on one side and into the nucleus pulposus on the other. At their periphery they merge with the annulus. At the centre of the disc is the nucleus pulposus, consisting of soft resilient fibrocartilage. It is incompressible but deformable. The volume of a lower cervical disc is $1-1\cdot4\,cm^3$ while that of a lumbar disc is about $10\,cm^3$.

The annulus fibrosus is the strongest part and serves to transmit tension through the spine. Its attachments are also extremely strong and, both anteriorly and laterally, it merges with the anterior longitudinal ligament; the combined structure is so strong that the bone is much more likely to fracture than the combined ligament and annulus is to tear. The posterior longitudinal ligament is not as well developed as the anterior one and, in addition, the annulus structure is weaker posteriorly. There are no blood vessels in the intervertebral disc, nutrition being carried out through the cartilaginous plates, and where this fails, the intervertebral disc space narrows. It also alters with age and in both these states there is a reduction in water content. The normal function of the nucleus pulposus lies in its compressibility and this changes with dehydration.

The nucleus pulposus deteriorates first with loss of its substance leading to inability to absorb shocks, to narrowing of the intervertebral space, and eventually degeneration of the annulus. It is possible for adjacent vertebrae to slide upon the loose tissue in a degenerating disc and occasionally this is seen radiologically in the cervical region and sometimes in the lumbar region.

Degeneration of a disc

A degenerating disc bulges in all directions but those in the anterior and lateral directions are unimportant compared to bulging which occurs posteriorly, when it will encroach on the intervertebral foramina or the spinal canal, causing a prolapse or herniation of the intervertebral disc. In this situation it may press on nerve roots or the spinal cord. This is the soft disc.

Following degeneration of a disc, it no longer acts as a shock absorber and the vertebral body expands and mushrooms out under the influence of normal stresses. The transverse surface of the vertebral body develops a re-active sclerosis which is seen on radiography as a dense margin to the inter-vertebral disc space; outgrowths of bone develop at the edge of the inter-vertebral surface and transverse ridges or osteoarthritic bars arise and can press upon the spinal cord. Correspondingly, there may be osteophytes later-ally which compress nerve roots.

In the soft disc—which in effect is a rupture of the annulus fibrosus fol-lowed by protrusion of the nucleus pulposus—the protrusion can be in the midline, paracentrally or laterally. Midline protrusion may produce cord compression, paracentral protrusion can produce either cord compression or nerve root compression or even both, and a lateral protrusion will produce a nerve root compression. The type of symptoms the patient develops de-pends on the level in the spine at which this happens.

The common prolapse occurs in the posterolateral annulus fibrosus close to the intervertebral foramen. However, a prolapsed disc does not press upon the nerves passing through that particular foramen but on the lower nerve root. This is where the trapped root crosses the disc and descends under the next lamina to leave the spinal cord below that pedicle and lamina. If the disc prolapse is a very large one, it may press upwards on to the foramen and can affect that nerve root; this is uncommon except in the L5/S1 region where a large lateral disc can spread upwards towards the foramen and the L5 nerve root may be affected in addition to the S1 root.

An affected nerve root lies to one side or the other of the protrusion or it can lie on its apex. The nerve is tethered by the thecal sheath where it leaves the spinal theca at the axilla; if the prolapse presses here, the nerve is com-pletely fixed and is unable to slide out of the way. Normally, relief of pain is obtained by the nerve root slipping from the apex of the bulge and this is probably how mobilization and manipulation works but the great danger of this treatment is that the prolapse increases in size and may develop into a detached sequestrum.

The cervical disc

In the cervical region the bodies of the cervical vertebrae articulate at their edges with the discs forming the neurocentral or Luschka's joint; osteo-phytes frequently develop here and then lie immediately anterior to the cervi-cal nerve root and medial to the vertebral artery. As spondylosis deformans accentuates the normal curves of the spine there is hyperextension of the cervical spine with shortening. This shortening is due to loss of intervertebral disc substance; the discs normally provide about one-quarter of the total length of the spine and as a result of the shortening the laminae tend to over ride each other and, most important, the ligamentum flavum bulges pos-teriorly into the spinal canal and diminishes its capacity.

Normally all these patients complain of pain radiating down the arm due to compression of the nerve root. Ruptures of the fifth and sixth cervical discs produce pain in the lateral aspect of the upper arm and the dorsum of the forearm. A protrusion lying between C5 and C6 vertebrae produces compression of the cervical sixth nerve root, causing pain in the neck, shoulder, the medial border of the scapula, the lateral aspect of the arm and the dorsum of the forearm. There may also be numbness of the thumb and index finger and a mild weakness of the biceps muscle.

When the protrusion lies between C6 and C7 with compression of the seventh nerve root, the pain is very similar to that of the cervical sixth nerve root but the numbness will be in the index and middle fingers with marked weakness of the triceps muscle and the triceps jerk will be reduced or absent.

A protrusion between C7 and T1 gives pain in the neck, the medial border of the scapula, the anterior chest and the medial aspect of the upper arm and forearm. There is numbness of the little and ring fingers and there is marked, sometimes extreme, weakness of the wrist and hand.

The frequency of the cervical intervertebral disc lesions compared to lumbar intervertebral disc lesions is 1:25, with lesions of the cervical discs between C6 and C7 being three times as common as between C5 and C6. Protrusions between C4 and C5, and C7 and T1 are much less frequent.

When a transverse osteophytic bar (the hard disc) presses on the cord, a myelopathy may occur and this produces the signs and symptoms of cord compression in the lower limbs and body. The treatment of this condition depends on whether the changes produced can be relieved, whether further deterioration can be prevented, or whether the condition is inoperable.

Conservative measures immobilize the cervical spine, preventing flexion and extension movements which would cause intermittent ischaemia from indentation and deformation of the spinal cord. Skull traction can be used where myelopathy with severe neck pain and brachial neuralgia is present. This would normally be followed by immobilization with a collar.

If traction is unnecessary, a collar is valuable whilst physiotherapy, heat and mobilization will all help. Manipulation is sometimes used for stiffness and to provide a fuller range of movement but it must be used with great caution.

When the soft disc produces symptoms, surgical removal of the prolapsed intervertebral disc is carried out but when the symptoms are due to bony spondylosis and myopathy other types of surgery are necessary. The Cloward operation is an anterior approach through the disc space which allows the disc, any transverse bar and the foramen to be cleared out, followed by an anterior fusion. However, when a number of disc spaces need treating, a posterior approach and decompression may be used. In very severe cases a Cloward operation together with a posterior decompression may be necessary.

The thoracic disc

Although radiological degeneration of thoracic discs is seen frequently symptoms are uncommon. This is probably a result of the thoracic spine being less flexible than either the cervical or lumbar spine and therefore less likely to become strained.

Thoracic disc prolapses can be divided into three groups according to clinical signs. First is a cord compression syndrome; symptoms and signs develop from this, causing a progressive paraparesis with impairment of all types of sensibility associated with nerve root pain and a disturbance of sphincter action. Second is a progressive paraparesis which is usually painful, and third is a radicular type of pain producing girdle and intercostal symptoms.

These prolapsed discs are treated according to the compression syndrome produced by them and involves surgery in all but the third type which may settle with rest and immobilization.

The lumbar disc

Degeneration of a lumbar disc is the most common cause of low back pain and sciatica, being more common than all the other causes of low back pain. In 95 per cent of cases, the fourth or fifth lumbar disc, or both, are involved.

A large retropulsion of a lumbar prolapsed disc presses upon the cauda equina and produces weakness of the sphincters, with pain in the midline of the back, the posterior thighs and leg. Numbness occurs in the same distribution and also the perineum, extending into the legs and soles of the feet. Paralysis of the feet and of the sphincters may occur and the ankle jerk may be absent. Gross symptoms of this type are usually due to discs at L4 or L5 level and are usually produced by injury. Most lumbar disc protrusions have a history of a vigorous muscular effort previously; the commonest one is lifting a heavy weight with the spine flexed.

A prolapse between L3 and L4, producing pressure on the fourth nerve root, gives pain in the sacroiliac joint, the hip, the posterolateral aspect of the thigh and the anterior aspect of the leg. Numbness occurs on the anteromedial portion of the leg and there is weakness of extension at the knees. The knee jerk is decreased or absent.

A prolapsed disc between L4 and L5 presses on the fifth nerve root, producing pain in the sacroiliac joint, the hip, the posterolateral aspect of the thigh and leg with numbness in the lateral aspect of the leg or the dorsum of the foot, including the big toe. Dorsiflexion of the big toe and, sometimes, of the foot is weak. There is no change in the reflexes.

The L5/S1 disc compresses the first sacral root, producing pain over the sacroiliac joint, the hip, the posterolateral aspect of the thigh, the leg and the heel. Numbness is present on the lateral aspect of the leg and foot, including the lateral three toes. Weakness is uncommon but when present, plantar flexion of the foot and the great toe is reduced, while the ankle jerk is reduced or absent.

Treatment is usually conservative except for the massive retropulsion. Any disc lesion producing alteration in control of sphincters must be regarded as an emergency. Conservative treatment consists of total rest on a firm bed and large doses of analgesics. Bed rest should last three weeks and the patient should not be allowed to get up to go to the toilet. When the symptoms are milder, this vigorous conservative regimen may not be required, but in all cases exercises to strengthen the erector spinae muscles are necessary and the lifting of weights should not be carried out for at least three months.

Injections can be made into muscles in spasm, or extradurally to give complete relief of pain for a time. The use of epidural blocks combining a local anaesthetic (7 ml of 1 per cent lignocaine) with 120 mg methylprednisolone acetate (3 ml Depo-Medrone) is of value in about half the cases and can be repeated, bearing in mind the total dose of steroids given previously. It is best carried out at the level of the affected nerve root rather than given through the sacral hiatus. When the sacral hiatus is used a larger volume is injected (30–50 ml of $\frac{1}{2}$ per cent lignocaine) and this dilutes the steroid.

Radiological investigation

Radiological investigations are of great importance in elucidating difficult cases but in most cases a careful history and neurological examination will indicate the correct diagnosis during the first few attacks before surgical inter- ference has occurred. After surgery for the removal of a pathological retro- pulsed vertebral disc which is followed after an interval by further pain, the diagnosis is more difficult. Pain under these circumstances can be due to another prolapse at the same level if the disc space was not completely cleared and was then allowed to fuse. It can be due to a disc at another level of the spine, or to adhesions either from the surgery or from irritation due to radio- opaque contrast material such as iophendylate (Myodil). The use of metriza- mide has been a great advantage in radiculography as this water-based contrast dye is completely resorbed from the theca into the blood stream in about five hours. It can now be used at any level of the spinal cord quite safely, and it differs from iophendylate in that the latter shows up the thecal volume and any indentations into it; the metrizamide radiculogram not only shows this but also fills the dural extensions round the nerve roots. These then can be clearly seen and any disc protrusion present obstructing the filling of one or more of these dural extensions can be readily identified.

Iophendylate has been implicated in the marked adhesions which some- times develop after myelography. Metrizamide is not without problems, as severe headache can develop after its use in lumbar myelography; patients are advised to remain seated for five hours after its use, by which time it has been absorbed. It is now used at any level of the spinal theca, including the cervical region (Amundsen and Scalpe, 1975).

False results

There has always been a significant number of false results produced by the iophendylate myelogram, and although the incidence of these has been reduced by the introduction of the metrizamide radiculogram some are still present.

Other methods of demonstrating the prolapsed intervertebral disc have been sought and epidural venography, and discography have been developed.

Epidural venography

The epidural veins ascend in the spinal canal, passing over the posterolateral aspect of each intervertebral disc. A retropulsed vertebral disc, as it pro- trudes, presses on this vein and obstructs it. This obstruction can be demon- strated. The technique is difficult and involves catheterizing the left femoral vein and careful positioning so that contrast is injected into the epidural veins above and below the disc protrusion. The advantage is that it is very accurate and will show those lateral protrusions not demonstrated on radiculography.

Discography

In this technique contrast is injected into the substance of the disc and shows its internal structure. A rupture of the annulus allows the contrast to spread and the disc can be seen as normal or abnormal. There is still considerable controversy over its use because an injection can be made into a normal disc. The common indication for this procedure is to examine the disc above the level of a proposed fusion of the spine.

References

Amundsen, R., and Scalpe, I. O. (1975). Cervical myelography with a water soluble contrast medium (metrizamide). *Neuroradiology* **8**, 209–212.

Benn, R. T. and Wood, P. H. N. (1975). Pain in the back; an attempt to estimate the size of the problem. *Rheumatology and Rehabilitation* **14**, 121–128.

Brewerton, D. A. (1975). Histocompatibility and rheumatic disease. *Annals of the Rheumatic Diseases* Suppl. 1, 34.

Kellgren, J. H. (1949). Deep pain sensibility. *Lancet* **i**, 943–949.

Lawrence, J. S. (1977). *Rheumatism in Populations*. Chapter 8, p. 282. Heinemann, London.

Melzack, R. (1975). Prolonged relief of pain by brief, intense, transcutaneous somatic stimulation. *Pain* **1**, 357–373.

Melzack, R., Stilwell, D. M. and Fox E. T. (1977). Trigger points and acupuncture points for pain; correlations and implications *Pain* **3**, 3–23.

Travell, J. and Rinzler, S. H. (1952). The myofascial genesis of pain. *Postgraduate Medicine* **11**, 425–434.

10

The treatment of chronic pain

Principles

Patients suffering from chronic pain can be divided broadly into two groups: those who have a normal expectation of life and those who have a short expectation of life. There are two important differences between these two groups.

The first difference is in relation to the time available for normal recovery of the central nervous system from damage. Recovery from ablation of portions of the central nervous system can vary from six weeks to several years and this is most important practically, as excellent pain relief can be produced by destruction of central nervous pathways. The simplest method of carrying this out is to destroy a peripheral sensory nerve such as when the supraorbital nerve is destroyed completely by an injection of alcohol or by surgical avulsion. The area of skin of which this is the afferent nerve will become anaesthetic, but over a period of time this nerve regenerates and, as regeneration spreads at an approximate rate of 1 mm per 24 hours, after a finite time sensation returns. However, when sensation returns it does not initially recover perfectly and completely. It may not return with exactly the same sensitivity and accuracy as previously but, nevertheless, sooner or later some sensation will return. However, if not all the sensory nerve fibres have been destroyed, recovery may not take as long as this; e.g. neurolytic sybstances injected near, and sometimes into, nerves do not destroy all the nerve fibres. Even avulsion of a nerve, or the sectioning and removal of a portion of it, may not be effective because there may be an accessory nerve a short distance away (this can happen with the supraorbital nerve). In any case, some nerve fibres will always regenerate.

At the other end of the sensory nerve pathway any central damage to the nervous system, such as in a thalamotomy, occurs at a level where the representation of sensory information is essentially bilateral, and for this reason pain may reappear in from six to twelve weeks due to the opening up of collateral pathways.

The longest period of relief from destruction occurs in an intermediate position in the spinal cord in an anterolateral cordotomy, in which the anterior quadrant of the spinal cord is sectioned. This can relieve pain for anything up to ten years or more but most frequently sensation returns within two years (Nathan, 1963). Sensation does not usually return rapidly although it may do so; it usually returns slowly and gradually over a period of months. During the period of recovery following nerve section in the spinal cord, there is a peculiar, unpleasant quality to sensation in the area supplied until full sensation returns. Often it does not return, and the patient continues to appreciate all kinds of abnormal sensations.

For these reasons, patients with a normal expectation of life should not have any portion of their central nervous system damaged or destroyed because the end result to the patient may be a much more unpleasant and uncomfortable life than the initial one. It is always very difficult to persuade a chronic pain patient that he can be made worse, and the pain relief physician may have to act conservatively.

The second difference is in regard to the drugs which can be given to patients with a normal length of life compared to those given to patients with a short expectation of life. Patients who have a short expectation of life usually suffer from the pain of inoperable cancer, and their pain is continuous and becomes steadily more severe. When their pain is sufficiently severe to warrant it, these patients should be given narcotic drugs in sufficient strength, quantity and frequency to relieve their pain. It may be that pain can be so severe from this cause that only loss of consciousness can relieve it but often patients in this category are not given that relief which is their due because one or other of their physicians believes that they may become addicted. This is an ineffective argument and arises from inadequate thought. The problems of drug addiction are due essentially to social environment and patients who have a short life, of the order of two years or less, will not develop problems of a serious nature in this time. Even if they do become drug addicts, it will only be for a short period. It is the experience of the author and of many other workers in this field that patients who suffer chronic pain from cancer and have their pain relieved by a cordotomy, stop their narcotics immediately and do not get withdrawal symptoms. These patients relish the idea of once again having cerebral activity unclouded by narcotics.

On the other hand, unless the circumstances are the most exceptional, patients with a normal expectation of life should not be put on narcotic drugs. These are the patients who find the dose of any drug they are given insufficient and tend to increase the quantity and frequency of medication; they will probably become drug addicts if they are put on narcotic drugs. Patients of this type have conditions such as chronic sciatica, low back pain, and postherpetic neuralgia, none of which is life-threatening, though the quality of their lives is altered by the pain.

Cancer pain

Characteristics

The development of a cancer pain occurs in a progressive fashion. The pain is always present at one particular site, it is constant and gradually spreads in extent and increases in severity over a period of weeks or months. It never decreases in intensity and, furthermore, there is never any period free of pain. Even after medication there is always a background of pain which is often described as boring and aching in type and is not usually felt on the surface but deep inside the tissues. There are acute exacerbations which tend to last for hours.

When the pain is no longer mild it frequently wakes the patient from sleep. There is a characteristic history in relation to nocturnal pain. The patient takes some analgesic tablets, the pain is partly relieved and the patient goes to sleep. After a varying period, usually three to four hours, the patient wakes up with pain and takes more analgesic tablets. After a period of about half an hour, the pain settles down and the patient gets off to sleep again and the whole process is repeated. In severe types of pain the patient may repeat this process every few hours; often such patients adopt a special routine when they awake with pain because they know approximately how long it takes for their tablets to work; they fill the time with some routine occupation, such as having a cigarette, walking about the house if they are ambulant, having a cup of tea; but rarely do they sit and read.

Cancer pain is relieved by rest, and this applies particularly to cancer of the vertebrae, when a flexed position is usually the most comfortable one. But even cancer pain can often be relieved by simple analgesic drugs, when given regularly in full dosage and with a following dose of drug given sufficiently early for it to cover the pain that arises when the previous dose is wearing off. This allows the control of mild to medium pain for long periods of time. The important feature here is the regularity and easy availability of the drugs for the patient. In addition, help can be obtained by means of a hot-water bottle or electric warming pad which give relief by their heat. give relief by their heat.

One of the most obvious features of cancer pain is the demoralization of the patient as the disease progresses if the pain is not controlled. The patient becomes completely preoccupied with his pain and he neglects his previous interests, family, and personal habits and appearance. This type of demoralization also occurs in patients with vascular insufficiency in a limb (usually the leg) or in the dystrophies such as causalgia or phantom limb pain. All these patients give a withdrawn, sorrowful appearance and, above all, give the impression of suffering.

It has been mentioned previously that chronic pain is a combination of sensations with which is associated some degree of suffering and this mental attitude reaches a peak in the severe chronic pain of cancer. This type of unremitting pain produces such a burden of suffering that all other thoughts are driven out of the patient's mind and he is wearied and obsessed by his suffering. This is not an abnormal response to unremitting pain, it is the normal one; and when the pain is relieved, a return to his previous personality is achieved almost instantaneously.

There is one other problem which arises when the patient has previously been treated for cancer in radical fashion and then a year or two later develops pain. Treatment depends on whether the pain is due to recurrent local spread of the disease, to a secondary cancer or is unrelated to the earlier disease.

For example, it is often particularly difficult to determine the cause of recurrent perineal pain in someone who has had an abdominoperineal resection, as some of these patients develop pain from scarring or adhesions and it may not be possible to solve the problem by means of biopsy, x-ray changes, or the development of a palpable growth, for many months. In most cases it is possible to decide this question on the patient's sleep pattern at night; an alteration of sleeping habit to that mentioned previously for cancer suggests a recurrence of the disease.

Non-malignant pain

Characteristics

Patients with a normal expectation of life and chronic pain are among the most persistent visitors to the general practitioner's surgery and to the out-patient departments of hospitals. Despite protestations of their pain being so severe that it is 'an agony', or 'a torture', they do not show any of the signs of demoralization seen in cancer patients. For instance, someone with a post-herpetic neuralgia may go for years without alteration to his personal habits or his hobbies, or of his interest in his family. His nutrition is good and he appears well. He does, however, over-react to his pain and his constant refrain to the doctor is, 'can I have more of the drug?' or 'can I have a more powerful drug?'.

The history of medication with these patients also has a common pattern. A new drug is prescribed for them and for a week, or perhaps two weeks, they report great benefit from it. On the third week the benefit is not quite as great, and they suggest an increase in dose. In the fourth week, or thereabouts, they want much more of the drug or something more powerful; the whole process then repeats itself. Eventually, having run through the whole gamut of analgesic agents, they remain unsatisfied with whatever medication is given to them and are always demanding something more powerful.

How should these patients be treated? The answer to this question is a very personal one, as most doctors will refuse this type of patient addictive drugs, while a substantial minority will give narcotic drugs, believing that one of the doctor's functions is to relieve pain and that it is not ethical to refuse potent drugs to a person in pain. The author takes his stand with the former group, believing that to prescribe addictive drugs to a patient with a long-term non-malignant pain problem will always result in addiction in susceptible patients. The majority may well not become addicted but I have seen too many who have to dismiss the danger lightly. The fashion in which operant conditioning (described in Chapter 5) can alter someone's attitude to his pain shows that a patient with years of conditioning to painful behaviour can be retrained to more socially accepted ways. It must be emphasized once again that pain does not kill, although the patient may be extremely miserable because of it; therefore, there is no point in adding to the patient's misery by allowing him to become drug addicted as well.

Nevertheless, some useful non-addictive drugs can, and should, be used regularly, as they reduce the level of pain although they are unable to eliminate it. Despite its dangers, aspirin is still the common choice of the patients themselves, and it is rare indeed for them to visit a doctor with a painful condition without first trying an aspirin drug. Between two and three tons of aspirin are used per day in Britain (i.e. upwards of 8 million tablets); if it were not for its irritant gastric effects, it would be a very good mild analgesic indeed.

The three effects of aspirin—analgesic, antipyretic and anti-inflammatory—are a powerful combination, and it is particularly useful in any condition where there is local damage and irritation. This is usually known as the anti-prostaglandin effect although it is accepted that aspirin does not produce this effect direct but prevents the production of the prostaglandins which normally sensitize the tissues to the action of bradykinin. The recently introduced drug diflunisal (Dolobid), an analogue of aspirin, has a reduced incidence of side effects; it has no effect on bleeding time and does not produce tinnitus. It has an analgesic, antipyretic and anti-inflammatory action, with a prolonged activity. Its length of action is at least 8 hours and up to 12 hours. It is available in 250 mg capsules for an initial dose of 500 mg (two capsules) and thence one capsule twice per day. This dose can be safely doubled. If the results of widespread use of this drug support these claims, it should be extremely useful in the chronic pain field.

Aspirin (and, presumably, Diflunisal), is effective for bone pain and can be tried even with bone pain produced by carcinoma metastases. In those conditions where a stronger anti-inflammatory action is required, then indomethacin (Indocid), ibuprofen (Brufen) or naproxen (Naprosyn) can be given. Of these, indomethacin is the most potent and naproxen the least potent; this also relates to the descending order of incidence of complications—which are mainly gastric. When patients develop gastric complications or already have gastric disease, or when there is no need for a peripheral anti-inflammatory action, paracetamol is the drug of choice. The benefit of both a salicylate and paracetamol can be obtained with benorylate (Benoral), which is an ester of the two substances and does not separate into its constituent parts until absorbed into the blood stream. In this way gastric irritation is avoided but not other complications of either drug. It is useful in musculoskeletal pain and in oestoarthritis and rheumatoid arthritis. A larger dose can be given by the suspension (10 ml b.d. containing 8·0 g) than by the tablets (2 tabs eight-hourly containing 4·5 g).

Drug therapy

Before concluding the discussion of the drugs to be used in chronic pain from non-malignant or malignant conditions, some general principles must be considered. To be useful, a drug must have an effective concentration at its site of action. If the concentration of drug falls below a critical level, it will have no action and yet there will be an appreciable quantity of the drug circulating in the blood. If a drug is injected intravenously, intramuscularly or subcutaneously, the whole of the dose is available for transport by the circulation.

However, transport is not a simple matter, as a dynamic equilibrium develops between plasma and tissue concentrations of the drug; to some extent this depends upon the blood supply of the tissue involved and so some tissues achieve a higher drug concentration earlier than tissues with a poor blood supply. In time, there is an equilibration between the tissues although those with a high lipid content will have a higher concentration. The ratio of the free to the bound form of the drug is constant and the drug level is prevented from falling by the transfer of drug from the sites on which they are reversibly bound. In time, the concentration of the drug falls because of its metabolism and excretion.

Most drugs are metabolized in the liver by enzymes and this is often affected by other drugs given at the same time. Barbiturates are particularly active in this respect and, when given, stimulate production of enzyme which is used in its own rapid breakdown. Other drugs which are metabolized by the same enzymes will also be broken down and this will occur more rapidly. In most cases the breakdown compounds produced by drug metabolism are less pharmacologically active than the parent compound and more easily excretable because they are more water-soluble. Very occasionally, metabolic alteration will increase pharmacological potency, as when codeine is demethylated to morphine.

Drugs given intravenously achieve their maximum plasma level almost immediately; when given subcutaneously or intramuscularly, a longer period of time is taken to do this and, indeed, because of the concomitant redistribution which occurs, the peak level is never as high as that by intravenous injection. Unfortunately, many drugs which absorb quickly and easily by parenteral injections are poorly absorbed by mouth. Narcotics come into this category; when absorbed from the alimentary tract, they pass into the portal system and through the liver where they may be detoxicated in part (first pass effect). Thus, larger doses and a slower action can be expected. It should be noted as a matter of interest that drugs administered by rectal suppositories are absorbed direct into the general circulation and do not pass through the portal circulation; therefore, their onset of action is rapid and they avoid the first pass effect which occurs with orally administered drugs.

The ideal of drug therapy is to administer the drug in such a way that the plasma concentration remains constant. It should remain constant above the level at which its activity begins but below the level at which further useful activity does not occur—this being the level above which undesired side effects are produced. Earlier in this chapter it has been mentioned that a succeeding dose of a drug should be given before the effect of a previous dose has worn off. What is implied by this is that, whether the drug is given parenterally or orally, it should be administered in such a way that the drug plasma concentration remains constant. The only method of maintaining concentration as constant as this, at the present time, is by the use of infusion pumps which give metered amounts of drug through an intravenous line. This technique is used to some extent in the Cardiff method of giving intravenous pethidine during childbirth. This device allows the mother to obtain pethidine on demand but prevents excessive use by an over-riding control which limits the frequency of the dose. The use of Entonox in childbirth is also a method of providing a fixed plasma concentration of an analgesic—in this case, nitrous oxide. The ideal drug would be one which is rapidly absorbed from the stomach without irritant effects, without side effects, without addiction and with one or two doses per 24 hours producing complete relief of the most intense pain. Unfortunately, there is no such drug available at present. Any discussion on how to prevent pain by medication assumes that this is possible and the evidence produced by hospices for the terminally ill (Saunders, 1978) shows that this is so, provided care and attention to regular doseage is made. It is simple to relieve pain by rendering the patient semi-conscious but since most patients want to take part in social activities, this degree of depression is acceptable only in the terminal stage. However, it must be recognized that, because of the danger of addiction, it is much more likely that patients with non-malignant pain—rather than those with malignant conditions—will not obtain complete relief.

The side effects of constipation, nausea and vomiting, and respiratory and circulatory depression may appear and will need counter-medication in either group of patients.

In patients with a malignant condition the salicylates and other mild analgesics already mentioned can be used in the early stages but, as the condition progresses and pain increases, other stronger drugs will be necessary. There will be a steady progression through such compounds as dihydrocodeine tartrate (DF 118), dipipanone (Diconal), methadone (Physeptone), pentazocine hydrochloride (Fortral), dextromoramide tartrate (Palfium). If stronger action is required morphine can be given orally.

It should be noted that pentazocine and pethidine, although effective analgesics when given parenterally, are not particularly potent oral analgesics; dextromoramide is most effective in relieving pain but its action is relatively brief—only one to two hours—and therefore it is useful as an additional drug if breakthrough pain occurs. Methadone has a long plasma half-life and there is a tendency for it to accumulate if care is not taken in the way it is used. There are two other drugs which may be used at longer intervals than the others: levorphanol (Dromoran) and phenazocine (Narphen). These are satisfactory on a six-hourly frequency when the pain is not too severe. An effective drug with a long action by mouth is bezitramide; it has a long duration of action with a slow onset, and for this reason there is the danger of respiratory depression.

Most of the narcotic drugs mentioned have an abuse potential and hence all of them are potentially addictive. Pentazocine is the least addictive though it will undoubtedly produce addiction in a small percentage of patients. This is one of the opiate antagonist substances which has effects somewhere between the opiates on the one hand and the pure antagonists such as naloxone on the other. Further work continues to produce drugs which combine analgesic potency with a weak antagonist action and a low or no abuse potential. The drug which so far approaches this ideal most closely is pentazocine.

It is necessary to know what drugs one is giving. By this is meant not just the name of the particular drug but its relative effective quantity and frequency compared to other drugs prescribed. This is best done by converting oral narcotics into their approximate oral morphine equivalents. Thus dipipanone (Diconal: dipipanone plus cyclizine) 10 mg = 5 mg of morphine sulphate, papaveretum (Omnopon) 10 mg = 5 mg of morphine; levorphanol (Dromoran) 1·5 mg is equivalent to 8 mg of morphine, and phenazocine (Narphen) 5 mg is equivalent to 25 mg of Morphine (Twycross, 1978). It must be remembered that pain levels can decrease as well as rise, and during long-term use it may be reasonable to reduce a patient's narcotic drugs, allowing the drug dosage to be controlled by the intensity of the pain. Furthermore the diagnosis and treatment of a new pain in a patient with a terminal illness should be carried out in the same fashion as in a patient coming with a completely new pain, as it may not be caused by the original condition but may be due to a pressure sore or a tooth ache; for instance, a headache may be due to a cerebral secondary with raised intracranial tension and the treatment of this is by large doses of dexamethasone, not more analgesics.

Pain relief is only part of the problem with patients who are suffering from inoperable conditions. Agitation, anxiety and depression are common, and drugs to control these are very necessary. When a patient is agitated one of the phenothiazines may be useful, as they produce sedation, drowsiness and a sensation of relaxation. Some of this group, such as chlorpromazine, potentiate the analgesic effects of narcotics and some, such as methotrimeprazine, have an analgesic activity themselves. In addition, they are anti-emetic and anti-histaminic, and although they cause little respiratory depression themselves they can have additive effects with the narcotics. They may have hypotensive effects due to α-adrenergic blockade and they can produce jaundice and extrapyramidal reactions. They should not be used in large doses because they depress the social and mental activity of the patient.

Hypnotics such as barbiturates are used for the production of sleep but they can produce dependence if used for a long time. In large doses they depress respiration and circulation and generally it is preferable that they be replaced with other drugs.

Anxiety can be treated with a number of drugs which include tranquillizers, hypnotics and the benzodiazepines. The latter are excellent and diazepam (Valium) is most effective.

Depression is treated by the tricyclic compounds. Of these, amitriptyline (Tryptizol) is most useful but it takes a week or so to become effective. It should be given at night in doses of about 50 mg and the patient warned that there may be dry mouth, blurring of vision and unsteadiness of gait. Amitriptyline has a sedative effect as well as an antidepressive one and this helps to relieve anxiety.

When pain is due to depressive illnesses, it will respond rapidly to antidepressive medication and to very little else. Certain pain syndromes, of which post-herpetic neuralgia is a good example, have pain due to lesions affecting the nervous system and these respond to some extent to the phenothiazine drugs. The method by which they work is unknown but some substituted phenothiazines block substances involved in nervous transmission. These drugs in large doses can have an analgesic effect on their own, and a combination of a substituted phenothiazine such as fluphenazine hydrochloride (Moditen) 1 mg t.d.s. with amitripytiline (Tryptizol) 50–75 mg at night was recommended by Taub and Collins (1974). The dose of fluphena-zine should be kept below 4 mg daily, or sedation, hypotension and extra-pyramidal reactions occur.

Anticholinesterase drugs can potentiate and prolong the analgesic effects of narcotics and, in addition, can reduce the urinary retention and constipa-tion produced by morphine. Amiphenazole (Daptazole) and tetrahydroa-minacrine (THA) can be used to increase the analgesic activity of morphine.

Where spasticity from disseminated sclerosis and other spinal cord condi-tions exists with painful spasms, the drug baclofen (Lioresal) is effective. Baclofen is a derivative of GABA, which is present in the central nervous system in large quantities and is known to inhibit neurotransmission. Baclofen depresses spinal neurones, reducing mono- and polysynaptic reflexes. Clinically, it reduces muscle tone, clonus and spasm with little de-pression of the cerebral cortex. Orphenadrine citrate (Norflex) may be useful in spastic conditions. It has an action which is due to its atrophine-like effect on neural transmission; its side effects include anxiety states, blurring of vision and dry mouth.

Summary

The purpose of drug therapy in the relief of pain is to allow the patient to lead as normal a life as possible. If at all possible, drugs should be given regularly, by mouth, and should be graded to the general level of pain. Persist-ence with weak analgesics or narcotics in severe pain is a waste of time and the patient suffers while the physician prepares himself to give a stronger narcotic. Conversely, if the pain level should fall there should be no hestita-tion in reducing the strength and quantity of the drugs and allowing the patient to benefit. Adjuvant drugs will be necessary, partly to increase the analgesic effect of the narcotic. This may be effected by adding an anti-cholinesterase such as neostigmine 15 mg or a phenothiazine, benzdiazepine, or a tricyclic compound. Sleep is important to these patients, particularly sleep which takes place at the same time as other people, so part of the daily intake of chlorpromazine or diazepam can be given at night. It must be remembered that patients with severe pain will need medication through the night and this should be easily accessible. The complications of urinary reten-tion and constipation should be dealt with.

When the patient has a normal expectation of life, a regimen with increas-ing doses of narcotics as time goes by cannot be entertained. Agitation, anxiety and depression are dealt with and such physical treatments as are available should be tried and the patient maintained with analgesic drugs. Pentazocine may be very useful if it relieves the patient's condition, as it has a very low abuse potential with mild narcotic effects although, as mentioned, it is addictive to a slight extent. Discontinuance of this drug after long admin-istration will cause only mild withdrawal symptoms. It can produce sedation and respiratory depression but these are minor disadvantages and it is always worth a trial in those patients in whom it does not produce psychotomimetic effects. Patients with a normal expectation of life who do not respond to the milder drugs or active measures ultimately either have to learn to live with their pain or they can try one of the relaxing techniques such as alpha feedback, Zen Buddhism, or electrical stimulation.

New drugs

There are two recent additions to the analgesic pharmacopoeia. They are both (like pentazocine) said to be non-addictive. They are nefopam (Acupan; 30 mg tablet, 20 mg injection) and buprenorphine (Temgesic; 0·3 mg injection, sublingual tablet). Nefopam is unrelated chemically or pharmacologically to the benzomorphan narcotic drugs usually used, being a benzoxazocine heterocyclic compound with a six-hourly dose. Temgesic is a powerful agonist–antagonist narcotic drug with an eight to twelve hour dose. An effective oral form is being sought and may be marketed soon.

Acupan may prove useful in the long life expectancy patient if it proves to be as non-addictive as claimed.

References

Saunders, C. (1978). *The management of terminal disease.* Edward Arnold, London.

Taub, A. and Collins, W. F. (1974). Observations on the treatment of denervation dysesthesia with psychotropic drugs. In: *Advances in Neurology*, Vol. 4, pp. 309–315. Ed. by J. J. Bonica. Raven Press, New York.

Twycross, R. G. (1978). Lecture delivered at a course on the Relief of Pain, Salford University, March 1978.

Further reading

Foldes, F. F. (1974). The role of drugs in the management of intractable pain. In: *Relief of Intractable Pain*, pp. 222–243. Ed. by M. Swerdlow. Excepta Medica, London and Amsterdam.

Williams, N. E. (1977). The role of drug therapy. In: *Persistent Pain*, Vol. 1, pp. 238–252. Ed. by S. Lipton. Academic Press, London and New York.

11

Electrical neuromodulation

If the gate theory is correct, then an increased input into the spinal cord from the large myelinated fibres should reduce the sensation of pain. In 1967 Wall and Sweet stimulated electrically their own infraorbital nerves and demonstrated decreased sensation in the infraorbital nerve distribution. They showed that stimulating the primary afferent neurone produced pain relief.

Since then it has been shown that stimulation of the dorsal column will also produce the same type of pain relief (Shealy, 1975) by antidromic conduction, and that stimulation of the brain will also produce pain relief. This technique goes under the comprehensive name of neuromodulation.

Intractable pain is not easily controlled by drugs or blocking techniques for any length of time and therefore the use of transcutaneous electrical stimulation can most logically be used for relief of chronic pain. It can indeed be used for acute pain, and trials of transcutaneous methods continue to evaluate its use in, for instance, the relief of postoperative incisional pain (Hymes *et al.*, 1974). In this method, strips of sterile electrodes are placed on each side of the wound and transcutaneous electrical stimulation is passed between them continuously in the postoperative period.

There are many varieties of electrical devices for transcutaneous stimulation but they usually have a square wave pulse, with the pulse width, the frequency and the power variable. Some devices fix one of these parameters (usually the pulse width), but on occasion both pulse width and frequency are fixed. Some transcutaneous stimulators provide for more than one pair of electrodes, and hospital models which are larger in size may provide for the treatment of two patients at one time and for the measurement of the various parameters.

Those models designed solely for patient use are small, can be easily hidden on the person, and may have a clip so that they can be attached to a belt or other article of clothing. These machines are battery powered so there is a limited period of activity, which can be overcome by using rechargeable batteries. Fortunately, most patients do not need maximum power and low outputs give very long battery lives. The voltage used varies from apparatus to apparatus but is within the range 0–70 volts. The frequency lies between 0 and 120 Hz, with the most commonly used range being 30–60 Hz. The pulse width is up to 500 μs. In effect, alteration of the pulse width tends to behave in similar fashion to an alteration of power, though there are a few patients whose pain relief seems to depend on careful adjustment of this control.

Many types of electrodes are used, from those similar to e.c.g. electrodes to flexible carbon ones. There is no doubt that the latter are much the best and are less likely to produce burns. All electrodes are used with electrode jelly and are held in place with adhesive tape. Some patients are sensitive to the adhesive used and care must be taken, as the electrode is kept against the skin for very long periods and a contact rash can occur.

Technique

The technique of using transcutaneous stimulators essentially entails teaching patients to use them themselves in their home and place of work. The electrodes are placed so that the stimulation occurs through or on the painful area. If the painful area is too tender for the electrodes to be placed directly on it, they are used at its periphery, and if possible the peripheral sensory nerve supplying that area is stimulated. The patients are told that the optimum position of the electrodes has to be found by trial and error, and they or their relatives are shown how to slide the electrode over the skin to do this. If an electrode is lifted off the skin, the apparatus must be switched off before the electrode is replaced or an electric shock will result.

Normally a pleasant, non-painful, tingling in the painful region is what is required and it will relieve pain when the method is going to be effective. Usually within 5 or 10 minutes the patient knows whether or not it is going to be successful (Nathan and Wall, 1974). Next, the frequency control is used and the patient is asked to find which is the most comfortable rate to use. Usually it is around 50 Hz, and when this has been adjusted the pulse width is altered. The pulse width seems to behave as another power control but about 10 per cent of patients do find this adjustment helps (Glynn, 1977).

Those who respond satisfactorily on a first stimulation need a stimulator to try regularly for long periods at home and, if possible, at work. This is the only way of finding out whether a particular patient will respond satisfactorily over a prolonged period. The method may not relieve pain completely but may be effective when combined with other methods. The patient must be told that the same setting of the controls will not always produce the same effect and may need altering from day to day.

The length and frequency of each stimulation session vary from patient to patient but at least three daily sessions of one hour are needed. Long (1977) suggests beginning with two to four hours of stimulation three to four times per day. Some patients stimulate all day, others before sleeping and some intermittently during the day. Each patient has to find the best combination to suit himself. The method of selection of suitable patients varies with each doctor but the simplest and most logical method is to give a trial of transcutaneous stimulation to anyone whose pain has a cutaneous element. It is logical to do this because transcutaneous stimulation is a non-invasive method which can be used on any patient, however ill, without risk, and theoretically its effect should not alter with time. In fact, it does alter with time; figures from the USA give 60 per cent initial improvement, falling subsequently to 30 per cent. In post-herpetic neuralgia, Nathan and Wall (1974) had approximately 30 per cent of patients obtaining good relief, with a few being cured after prolonged stimulation over two years. Experience in the Centre for Pain Relief in Liverpool is not as conclusive. About the same proportion of patients receives relief as one would anticipate in placebo reactors (Evans, 1974). However, it is believed (as stated also by Glynn) that if pain relief lasts for a year, it is unlikely to be dependent on a placebo response.

The conditions treated by transcutaneous stimulation include low back pain, post-amputation pain, postoperative scar pain and post-herpetic neuralgia.

Dorsal column stimulation (DCS)

This is the name given to neuromodulation applied to the first neurone fibres in the posterior columns of the spinal cord (Shealy, 1975). In this method the electrodes are placed close to the posterior columns of the spinal cord and are stimulated by current with similar characteristics as those used for transcutaneous stimulation. The posterior columns contain a high percentage of large nerve fibres and are selected for this reason. Originally, electrodes were implanted surgically and either fixed inside the dura or an artificial pocket was made in the dura by splitting it and the electrode sutured into that. A later method was to insert a long epidural electrode by means of a Tuohy needle. It could be left *in situ* for a few days while an extended test of stimulation was carried out. At the Centre for Pain Relief such electrodes have been left in place for months in some patients. An extension of this method is to insert two epidural electrodes and bring them out subcutaneously about 15 cm from the midline. If the test stimulation over 24 hours or so is satisfactory, these electrodes can be cut short at the sterile portion subcutaneously, connected up to a receiver which is then left beneath the skin, and in this way an open operation is avoided.

In those patients whose pain is confined to a single peripheral nerve, electrodes can be implanted direct on to the nerve instead of the dorsal columns. The efficacy of the method can be forecast as in DCS by an electrode temporarily inserted, in this case, on to the nerve. The value of implanted peripheral nerve electrodes has been evaluated over many years and it is one of the most reliable methods of neuromodulation available (Long, 1977).

All implanted electrodes, whether for DCS, nerve, or brain stimulation, have a receiver attached to the electrode by buried wires. The receiver is placed subcutaneously at a convenient position. The patient then positions the aerial of a small pocket-sized radiotransmitter over the receiver and, in this way, electrical stimulation is transferred from the transmitter to the electrode.

Many thousands of DCS electrodes have been inserted in the USA but there have been problems, mostly due to poor selection of patients. The overall success rate is about 60 per cent and this is not sufficiently encouraging to offset the major surgery involved. However, it is most likely that this figure would be considered satisfactory for the percutaneous epidural method and that technique is now being re-evaluated. At the Centre for Pain Relief in Liverpool, a careful evaluation is made of potential DCS patients. The tests used involve abrasion of accessible nerves supplying the affected part; stimulation by transcutaneous stimulation; acupuncture; and injection of hypertonic saline into the dermatomal interspinous ligament. The first increases pain and, in a phantom limb pain, will exacerbate it markedly, while the last three will improve pain. The normal history, examination and treatments are also used and the final evaluation also includes the effect of prolonged epidural stimulation with tingling obtained in the distribution of the painful area, associated with relief of the pain (Miles *et al.*, 1974).

The second and third neurone

These neurones are stimulated at the specific sensory thalamic nuclei, or in the intralaminar nuclei of the thalamus, or in the sensory part of the posterior internal capsule (Hosobuchi, Adams and Rutkin, 1973, 1975). These methods have been used to relieve pain mainly of central origin such as anaesthesia dolorosa of trigeminal nerve distribution, but they can be used for organic pain, which is not controlled by a DCS, or where a DCS cannot be implanted because of technical reasons.

The flexible wire electrode is implanted at the selected target by a stereotactic procedure using a stereotactic frame in the standard fashion. A relatively small number of these electrodes have been implanted because of the difficult technical problems involved—of which two are most important. First, the exact position for the electrode has to be found since the stereotactic method is not quite accurate enough to allow for the normal variation of brain structures, and, secondly, there are problems in fixing the electrode in position.

The problems are overcome by using a compound electrode with multiple outlets. This electrode is inserted and exteriorized. Over some days various combinations of the outlets are tested for pain relief and these correspond to different stimulation sites near the tip of the electrode. When the best one is found, it is connected to a receiver button and the electrode is buried. Stimulation then takes place in identical manner to that in other implanted electrodes.

The cost of the equipment in either DCS or brain stimulation is approximately £1000.

References

Evans, F. J. (1974). The placebo response in pain reduction. In: *Advances in Neurology*, Vol. 4, pp. 289–296. Ed. by J. J. Bonica. Raven Press, New York.

Glynn, C. J. (1977). Electrical stimulation for pain relief. *British Journal of Clinical Equipment*, July, 184–189.

Hosobuchi, Y., Adams, J. E. and Rutkin, B. (1973). Chronic thalamic stimulation for the control of facial anesthesia dolorosa. *Archives of Neurology* **29**, 158–161.

Hosobuchi, Y., Adams, J. E. and Rutkin, B. (1975). Chronic thalamic and internal capsule stimulation for control of central pain. *Surgical Neurology* **4**, 91–93.

Hymes, A. C., Raab, D. E., Yonehiro, E. G., Nelson, G. D. and Printy, A. L. (1974). Acute pain control by electrostimulation. A preliminary report. In: *Advances in Neurology*, Vol. 4, pp. 761–767. Ed. by J. J. Bonica. Raven Press, New York.

Long, D. M. (1977). Electrical stimulation for the control of pain. *Archives of Surgery* **112**, 884–888.

Long, D. M. and Hagfors, N. (1975). Electrical stimulation in the nervous system. *Pain*, Vol. 1, **2**, 109–123.

Miles, J. B. (1977). Stimulation for the relief of pain. In: *Persistent Pain*, pp. 140–146. Ed. by S. Lipton. Academic Press, London and New York.

Miles, J., Lipton, S., Hayward, M., Bowsher, D., Mumford, J. and Molony, V. (1974). Pain relief by implanted electrical stimulators. *Lancet* **i**, 777–779.

Nathan, P. W. and Wall, P. D. (1974). Treatment of post-herpetic neuralgia by prolonged electrical stimulation. *British Medical Journal* **3**, 645–7.

Shealy, C. N. (1975). Dorsal column stimulation. *Surgical Neurology* **4**, 142–146.

Wall, P. D. and Sweet, W. H. (1967). Temporary abolition of pain in man. *Science* **155**, 108–109.

12

Acupuncture

Much has been written about acupuncture and whether or not it is valuable in a modern context. There is, however, no doubt at all that a proportion of patients can be operated upon under its influence and that it is useful in some types of pain relief (Kaada et al., 1974).

Acupuncture is an ancient Chinese system of medicine where a needle pierces the skin to a greater or lesser depth and is left there for a time. During this time it may be rotated or stimulated in some other fashion and is said to produce certain effects. It must be pointed out that acupuncture is a system of medicine in which the patient is observed and examined, a diagnosis is made and therapy instituted. The explanations given by the ancient Chinese to explain how acupuncture works should be regarded merely as the attempts of primitive scientists to explain observed phenomena in the words of the time. Thus, classical Chinese acupuncture uses the concept of the world being divided into the five elements of wood, fire, earth, metal and water and this is combined into their theories. They also bring into their system the idea of a life force or 'a something' which penetrates everything in the heavens and the earth. These beliefs had their counterparts in early European ideas of the ether which pervaded all things, and there was also a European idea of four elements of fire, earth, air and water.

The Chinese have formulated their ideas into universal laws of Yin and Yang, the meridians which are lines around the body where the life force flows, and acupuncture points at which particular effects can be obtained (Fig. 12.1). The decision as to which meridian and which acupuncture point should be used, depends on experience and the pulse diagnosis. Palpation of the radial pulses enables a properly trained acupuncturist to decide the correct positions for the acupuncture needles. The purpose of needling is to correct an abnormal flow of the life force into a normal flow and thus improve the diseased condition.

A great deal of importance is attached to what is talled 'take'. When an acupuncture needle is inserted to the correct depth, a sensation called 'take' is felt by the patient. This is a numb sensation which occurs within a few seconds and spreads from the site of acupuncture. The Chinese attach great importance to this and if, for instance, 'take' does not appear in a patient having acupuncture for operative intervention, then acupuncture is abandoned for that particular patient. Experimental work has been taking place on this particular aspect and it appears that 'take' is not necessary for analgesia to develop.

Very different figures are reported in respect of the frequency of treatment within China, depending on the authority quoted. Initially for acupuncture anaesthesia, a multiplicity of points was used but frequently nowadays it is reduced, often to the absolute minimum. Further, for some medical conditions a patient is seen and treated daily for a week or two; Kaada *et al.*, (1974) mention treatment for psychiatric conditions which involve three treatments per day for 30 minutes each time.

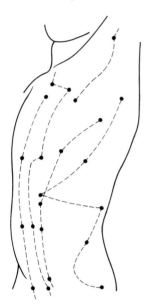

Fig. 12.1   Meridians and acupuncture points.

What, then, is the physiological position with regard to acupuncture? There is no doubt that acupuncture can relieve pain to some extent including acute pain in surgery. However, witnesses of these techniques in China have come to a number of conclusions. First, acupuncture appeared to be given in combination with large doses of hypnotic and analgesic drugs and, secondly, acupuncture in surgery was not used as frequently as the news media led one to believe; although in 1968 it was used in nearly 60 per cent of all operations in some hospitals in China, by 1972 this figure had dropped to about 20 per cent and in 1973 was less than this. Bonica in 1974 reported that some hospitals gave a percentage of only 5 or 6.

The success rate is said to be 85 to 90 per cent for most types of operation but the criteria of success in China appeared to be very different from those accepted in the West. Pain relief to our standards occurred in, at most, one-third of the patients operated upon using acupuncture analgesia and this itself was only a small percentage of the total number of operations. Nevertheless, on occasion a patient would have a complete operation of a kind which usually produced severe pain using nothing but acupuncture analgesia (Wall, (1975) personal communication).

Various theories have been advanced to explain acupuncture analgesia, and the traditional Chinese explanation has been touched on briefly. There are two main theories: one based on neurophysiological data, the other believing that the pain is relieved by psychophysiological mechanisms.

The neurophysiological explanations certainly suggest the involvement of a nervous mechanism in acupuncture analgesia. The simplest way of regarding this is to believe that acupuncture is another form of peripheral nerve stimulation, of the same general nature as transcutaneous peripheral nerve stimulation, and that the analgesic effect is similar to that produced by such stimulation. If the nerves innervating the acupuncture site are blocked, then acupuncture analgesia will not develop as expected. Similarly, acupuncture analgesia will not develop on the affected side in hemiplegic patients. The type of analgesia produced depends to some extent on the rate of stimulation. Acupuncture analgesia requires rather strong electroacupuncture which causes jerky movements of the muscles just below the patient's pain tolerance level. It appears that this type of activity stimulates deep pressure receptors and muscle stretch receptors, and this will produce analgesia. It is, incidentally, very similar to the technique, used in physiotherapy, of deep connective tissue massage. There is another mechanism since acupuncture analgesia can be produced by a low frequency stimulation of about 1–2 Hz, and this type of analgesia appears to develop in a more widespread fashion. This is the type of stimulation used for surgical acupuncture and it produces a gradual increase in the pain threshold in the course of 20–30 minutes. This is the time scale that is usually used in surgical acupuncture. High frequency stimulation causes an immediate and short-lasting effect which is strictly segmental, whereas the low frequency stimulation in the same patient has an effect that comes on gradually and outlasts the stimulation for several hours. This slow time of onset suggests that a humoral chemical factor is involved, and various cross-circulation experiments have shown that acupuncture analgesia developed over a period of 30 minutes can be transferred from one animal to another (Takeshige, Luo and Kamada, 1976). It is not known what this humoral factor is, but it is known that giving large doses of reserpine 24 hours before acupuncture increases the analgesic effect and this suggests that a substance such as serotonin might be liberated. It has also been shown that when acupuncture analgesia has been developed, naloxone will antagonize this effect (Mayer, Price and Rafii, 1977). The possible relation to the endogenous opiates is obvious.

The psychological factors which are considered to be effective in acupuncture analgesia are those of attention and anxiety. There is no doubt that acupuncture does have a calming effect, and many patients who have acupuncture treatment return after the first treatment mentioning that they were so relaxed and tired when they got home that they went to bed and slept for many hours. Acupuncture analgesia has also been explained on the basis of hypnotic suggestion or even a placebo effect. There is no doubt acupuncture analgesia, as any form of medical treatment, is greatly influenced by psychological factors (Chapman, Wilson and Gehrig, 1976; Hossenlopp, Leiber and Mo, 1976).

It would appear, therefore, that acupuncture analgesia does develop and that in clinical practice it can be used as a non-invasive simple method of relieving pain. In the author's experience, it is particularly useful in chronic migraine patients who do not respond to any of the normal treatments available; after they have been fully investigated to exclude neurological disease, acupuncture will produce relief in about two-thirds of them to the extent of a reduction of two-thirds in both the pain and the frequency of attacks. There will, of course, be some patients whose migraine is completely relieved and a few patients whose migraine appears to be made worse.

References

Bonica, J. J. (1974). Acupuncture anesthesia in the Peoples Republic of China. *Journal of the American Medical Association* **229**, 1317–1325.

Chapman, R. C., Wilson, M. E. and Gehrig, J. D. (1976). Signal detection evaluation of the effects of acupuncture on the perception of painful dental stimulation. In: *Advances in Pain Research and Therapy*, Vol. 1, pp. 775–779. Ed. by J. J. Bonica and D. Albe-Fessard. Raven Press, New York.

Hossenlopp, C. M., Leiber, L. and Mo, B. (1976). Psychological factors in the effectiveness of acupuncture for chronic pain. In *Advances in Pain Research and Therapy*, Vol. 1, pp. 803–809. Ed. by J. J. Bonica and D. Albe-Fessard, Raven Press, New York.

Kaada, B., Hoel, E., Leseth, K., Nygaard-Østby, B., Setekleiv, J. and Stovner, J. (1974). Acupuncture analgesia in the People's Republic of China. *Tidsskrift for den Norske Laegeforening* **94**, 417–442.

Mayer, D. J., Price, D. D. and Rafii, A. (1977). Antagonism of acupuncture analgesia in man by the narcotic antagonist naloxone. *Brain Research* **121**, 368–372.

Takeshige, C., Luo, C. P. and Kamada, Y. (1976). Modulation of E.E.G. and unit discharges of deep structures of brain during acupuncture stimulation and hypnosis of rabbits. In: *Advances in Pain Research and Therapy*, Vol. 1, pp. 781–785. Ed. by J. J. Bonica and D. Albe-Fessard. Raven Press, New York.

Further reading

Chaitow, L. (Ed.) (1976). *The Acupuncture Treatment of Pain*. Oxford University Press, Oxford.

Mann, F., Bowsher, D., Mumford, J., Lipton, S. and Miles, J. (1973). Treatment of intractable pain by acupuncture. *Lancet* **ii**, 57–60.

Mann, Felix (Ed.) (1971). *Acupuncture, the ancient Chinese art of healing*. Heinemann, London.

Mann, F. (Ed.) (1972). *An Atlas of Acupuncture: points and meridians*. Heinemann, London.

National Health and Medical Research Council of Australia (1974). *Report on Acupuncture*. Australian Government Publishing Service, Canberra.

Nogier, P. F. (Ed.) (1972). *Treatise of Auriculotherapy*. Maisonneuve, Moulins-les-Metz, France. (Details of an English translation are available from Maisonneuve.)

Wu Wei-p'ing (Ed.) (1962). *Chinese Acupuncture*. Translated and adapted by J. Lavier and P. M. Chancellor. Health Science Press, Rustington, Sussex.

Zhang Jin-an (Ed.) (1962). *The Yellow Emperors Book of Acupuncture*. Shanghai Scientific and Technical Publishing House. Peking.
    (1973). Translated by Henry C. Lu. Academy of Oriental Heritage, Vancouver, Canada.

13
Hypnosis

Hypnosis can relieve pain completely in patients who are highly suggestible but, because these form a small percentage of the population, it is more realistic to use hypnosis as an adjuvant analgesic. The induction of hypnosis is a straightforward and simple procedure, usually taking only a few minutes. The patient is asked to concentrate his attention and to think about his eyes and body getting heavy, and to allow himself to drift off to sleep. This sleep is a trance state in which he can clearly hear the operator's voice and carry out his instructions. When the trance is deep, instructions can be given that the body is insensitive to pain and eventually, in very susceptible patients, an operation can be carried out.

There is no clear physiological change on entering the hypnotic state and no obvious mechanism for suppressing pain. In fact, the patient can appear wide awake while hypnotized, after being given suitable commands or suggestions. However, there is one anomaly in that the patient does show changes in heart rate and respiration rate when, for instance, a normally painful procedure is carried out apparently painlessly in the hypnotized state. This type of phenomenon has raised questions about the reality of hypnotically induced anaesthesia, as it might be, for instance, that the subject is so eager to please the hypnotist that he just 'grins and bears the pain', the change in the physiological signs being the only sign of this happening.

It is possible in a deeply hypnotized patient to produce two changes: one is an anaesthetic arm, and the other is the ability to perform automatic writing with the non-anaesthetized arm on command but without the activity or sense of what is being written reaching consciousness.

The anaesthetized arm is stimulated, the patient is asked if he feels pain and the verbal reply is negative. He is then asked to show by the automatic writing what he feels and the answer is 'pain' (Hilgard, 1975). In similar fashion, automatic speaking can be developed so that in both these methods the patient acts as his own hidden observer. It appears that at cortical level the subject does appreciate pain but it is much less than that which would normally be experienced and there is no suffering involved.

The use of hypnoanalgesia can be extended to the treatment of postoperative pain or intractable cancer pain, but again only in those who are susceptible—less than 20 per cent of patients (Finer, 1972). Orne (1976), investigating the relationship between placebo effect and hypnotizability, showed that patients who were non-hypnotizable obtained pain relief equivalent to that of a placebo effect when they believed the procedure would be helpful, while those who were hypnotizable accepted the procedure and obtained a much more profound level of analgesia. The reason that about 90 per cent of all patients can obtain some relief of pain in dentistry under hypnosis, while it is known that susceptible patients form only 20 per cent of the population, is due to the patient becoming less anxious, allowing local injection without difficulty and being easier to manage. Thus, the suggestions of relaxation made during the hypnotic induction process tend to produce some general relaxation in all patients and they are also helped by the non-specific placebo effect—both these developing quite apart from those patients who achieve a hypnotic trance.

References

Finer, B. (1972). The use of hypnosis in the clinical management of pain. *Pain: basic principles; pharmacology; therapy* pp. 168–170. Ed. by J. P. Payne and R. A. P. Burt. Churchill Livingstone, Edinburgh and London.

Hilgard, E. R. (1975). The alleviation of pain by hypnosis. *Pain* **3,** 213–232.

Orne, M. T. (1976). Mechanisms of hypnotic pain control. In: *Advances in Pain Research and Therapy*, Vol 1, pp. 717–726. Ed. by J. J. Bonica and D. Albe-Fessard. Raven Press, New York.

14

Percutaneous cervical cordotomy

There are some methods of relieving pain which are very effective; these include the anterolateral cordotomy, the pituitary injection of alcohol (see Chapter 15) and the destruction of the nerves to the posterior intervertebral joints (the facet joint) (see Chapter 16). The first two of these methods are of value in the pain of intractable cancer when the patient has a reduced expectation of life, while the third method is useful in pain in the neck or back.

Surgical cordotomy

Ablative methods of pain relief are effective only when the patient does not live long enough for the sequelae to develop. Thus, although these methods can be used for any patient, they are best confined to those with a short expectation of life.

Surgical cordotomy was first carried out in 1912 (Spiller and Martin) and it consists of a surgical section of the anterolateral quadrant of the spinal cord, carried out under direct vision. If bilateral pain is to be relieved, then a laminectomy over one or two vertebrae is carried out and two spinal cord sections are made at different levels so that one is at the upper portion of the wound on one side and one at the lower portion of the wound on the other. This is to avoid possible postoperative difficulties from oedema, or haematoma compressing the spinal cord, and from disfunction.

For surgical cordotomy the anterolateral quadrant of the spinal cord is approached posteriorly so that the spinal cord has to be rotated somewhat for the surgeon to reach the anterior quadrant. It is possible that this twisting of the spinal cord interferes with its blood supply and has some part to play in the complications afterwards. These may include paresis and difficulty of micturition but they usually resolve spontaneously. In 1963, Mullan et al. used a radioactive tipped probe placed anterolaterally to the spinal cord through an intrathecal spinal needle at the C1–C2 level. This irradiated the spinal cord and destroyed part of it within about one week, producing analgesia of a lower quadrant of the body. If analgesia of the arm or upper quadrant of the body was required, then a longer period of irradiation had to take place. If the patient lived beyond two months or so, the radioactive effect continued, producing spreading destruction, causing paresis not only of the ipsilateral side but also of the opposite side.

In 1965 Mullan *et al.* aimed the spinal needle anterior to the dentate ligament, inserted an electrode into the spinal cord and then produced a traumatic lesion by means of a direct electric current. In the same year, Rosomoff *et al.* (1965), using a similar method of inserting the electrode, used a radiofrequency current (RFC)—i.e. a diathermy current—to heat coagulate the anterolateral quadrant. The direct current method took about 20 minutes to produce a lesion, whilst using the RFC method it occurred in about 30–60 seconds. Because of this speed of action the position of the electrode had to be determined accurately.

Lateral cordotomy

The RFC method is still used to-day but it has been refined to determine the exact position of the electrode in the spinal cord before ablation is commenced. Various electrodes are used and they can be made quite easily in the hospital workshop or can be bought ready made. The commercial ones have a matching spinal needle with an electrode which fits into the spinal needle in such a way that only the terminal 4 mm of the sharpened electrode tip projects from the end of the needle. The terminal 2 mm of the electrode is exposed, all the remainder being insulated. During insertion an impedance measurement (i.e. an electrical resistance measurement) is made through the electrode and this determines the end point of the insertion. The spinal needle is aimed anterior to the dentate ligament as before; as soon as the electrode is inserted, the exposed tip makes contact with cerebrospinal fluid and the resistance falls to a low level of about 200 ohms. When the tip is half in the spinal cord and half in the cerebrospinal fluid, the resistance is still low but slightly higher than at first—about 300 ohms. When the insulation of the electrode is flush with the surface of the spinal cord and is no longer in contact with cerebrospinal fluid, the resistance rises suddenly to over 800 ohms. This can be seen as a definite end point and insertion stops at that position. This avoids the electrode being inserted too deeply into the tissues.

Anteroposterior x-rays of the spinal cord through the open mouth will show the spinal needle and electrode in relation to the odontoid process. Normally, the centre of the odontoid process can be taken as the centre of the spinal cord, although it must be remembered that the spinal cord is not fixed rigidly and does move under the thrust of the electrode. The lateral x-ray shows the position of the electrode in relation to the C1–C2 vertebral space and if either air or iophendylate has been injected into the cerebrospinal fluid, the anterior border of the spinal cord or the dentate ligament, respectively, will be seen. The spinal needle is aimed at one or other of these with a measurement of 1–2 mm anterior to the dentate ligament or 3 mm or so posterior to the anterior border of the spinal cord. The next stage is to carry out stimulation studies, first at 2 Hz and later at 100 Hz. The stimulating

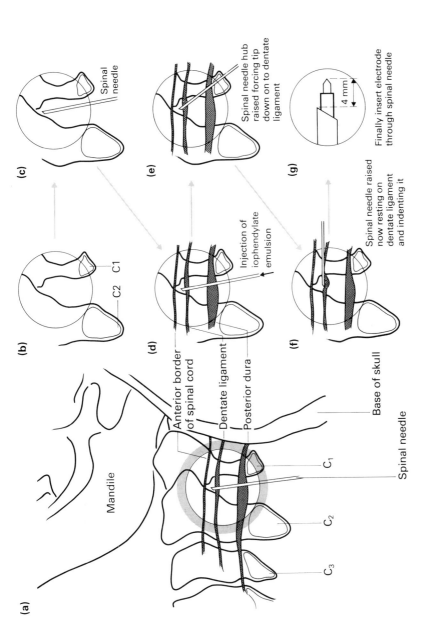

(a)

Mandile

Anterior border
of spinal cord

Dentate ligament

Posterior dura

C_1

C_2

C_3

Base of skull

Spinal needle

(b)

C2   C1

(c)

Spinal
needle

(d)

Injection of
iophendylate
emulsion

(e)

Spinal needle hub
raised forcing tip
down on to dentate
ligament

(f)

Spinal needle raised
now resting on
dentate ligament
and indenting it

(g)

4 mm

Finally insert electrode
through spinal needle

Fig. 14.1 Stages of percutaneous cervical cordotomy

current is applied through the electrode. At 2 Hz, with the electrode in the correct position, some of the nerve fibres from the anterior horn cells will be stimulated so that muscles on the ipsilateral side supplied by these fibres will contract regularly at 2 Hz. Usually the trapezius elevates the shoulder and/or the small muscles of the head produce a slight turning movement. If the muscles round the elbow, hand, body or leg contract, the electrode is inserted too posteriorly and is affecting the corticospinal fibres. Coagulation at this point will produce paresis and so the electrode position must be altered more anteriorly. It must be emphasized that every time an alteration in the position of the electrode takes place, the complete series of checks must be carried out: impedance measurement, anteroposterior and lateral x-rays, and, most important of all, stimulation studies.

When stimulation at 2 Hz is satisfactory, stimulation at 100 Hz can take place. This tends to stimulate sensory fibres rather than motor fibres and the patient usually has sensory hallucinations on the contralateral side of the body as the sensory fibres are crossed. When impedance measurement, x-ray evidence and stimulation studies show that the position is correct, a small RFC coagulation can be carried out to check where the analgesia will develop if full coagulation is carried out.

Coagulation involves the use of a special lesion generator, which in effect is a low-powered diathermy machine. Various commercial lesion generators are available and they usually contain, in the same machine, facilities for impedance measurement and for stimulation. Those machines which can also be used for thalamotomy, RFC distruction of the trigeminal nerve or facet rhizotomy will also have facilities for temperature control of the electrode tip. The cordotomy electrode is too small to include this facility. Most lesion generators produce enough heat to heat coagulate the anterolateral quadrant of the spinal cord in between 30 and 60 seconds at around 50 milliamps (mA). Coagulation occurs in one of two ways: either the current can be kept constant and the time varied so that, say, 50 mA is used for 2.5 seconds, 5 seconds, 7.5 seconds, and so on, checking the analgesia on the contralateral side and also any developing motor weakness on the ipsilateral side; or the time of, say, 30 seconds can be kept constant and the current altered so that it would be 30 seconds progressing from 20 mA, to 25 mA, then 30 mA, and so on, checks being made to test the analgesia on the one side and power on the other. If there is any decrease in strength on the ipsilateral side, then the position of the electrode must be reviewed very carefully. Motor power can be checked by asking the patient to hold his arm in the air and to bend the knee and dorsiflex the foot while coagulation is proceeding. In between coagulation the hand grip or dorsiflexion of the foot can be tested.

Coagulation is cautiously increased until analgesia, as shown by loss of sensation to pinprick, occurs on the correct side of the body. It can then continue until the painful area, plus a few segments higher or lower, has been completely covered by the analgesia. The process is repeated three times, using the same electrical parameters as in the last coagulation. Between each coagulation there should be an interval of one minute to allow for heat dissipation. This makes certain that all the sensory nerve fibres are destroyed. If all fibres are not destroyed, the patient will be sensitive in one small area and, if this was painful previous to the cordotomy, it will remain painful post-cordotomy. Provided care has been taken with the various tests and checks, there should be few complications. This method is extremely useful for patients with a unilateral pain which does not extend above the C5 dermatome. It is not satisfactory for higher lesions because the nerve fibres ascend three or four segments before crossing the spinal cord to the opposite anterolateral quadrant. Therefore, when the lesion is made at the C1–C2 space, analgesia on the opposite side will normally only occur up to and including C5. Occasionally, when there is a more rapid cross-over, fibres as high as C2 can be affected but this is unusual (Lipton, 1968; Ganz and Mullan, 1977).

Bilateral percutaneous cervical cordotomy

Bilateral percutaneous cervical cordotomies can be carried out but there are complications attached to this, as with any method of bilateral cordotomy carried out at the C1–C2 level. All bilateral cordotomies—even when a segment or two difference is made between the two levels on the two sides—will produce problems with micturition, and although these may improve, they do not disappear entirely. The percutanous cervical cordotomy from the lateral approach can be performed only at the C1–C2 space, and at this level in the spinal cord, the ascending and descending respiratory reticular fibres lie near the anterior horn cells. Thus, if a high level of analgesia is required, these fibres will tend to be destroyed. If they are destroyed on both sides of the spinal cord, a form of unusual apnoea can develop (Mullan and Hosobuchi 1968). The patient will be able to breathe voluntarily but has a reduced capacity for involuntary breathing with a tendency to stop breathing during sleep. The complete syndrome is known as the Ondine syndrome; Rosomoff (1969) has reported that about 4 per cent of patients with high bilateral cordotomies will develop this syndrome, of whom about half will die. The only treatment is to use artificial ventilation until recovery occurs. This condition can be avoided by carrying out a lateral cordotomy on one side and an anterior cordotomy on the other.

Anterior approach

The anterior cordotomy was developed by Lin, Gildenberg and Polakoff (1966) to avoid the problem of the Ondine syndrome in bilateral high cordotomies. In this method an approach is made at C5–C6 level from an anterior approach through a disc space. The needle enters the cerebrospinal fluid and the electrode is inserted into the anterolateral quadrant, the target being the same as that in the lateral approach. In the anterior approach the anterolateral quadrant is destroyed below the outflow of the phrenic nerve and, therefore respiratory problems do not arise (Lipton, Dervin and Heywood, 1974).

Posterior approach

A third method of carrying out a percutaneous cervical cordotomy is from a posterior approach with a fine electrode traversing the spinal cord from back to front. This is the method of Crue *et al.* (1970) and involves a stereotactic frame; it is more complicated than the methods already mentioned.

The main problem with a unilateral percutaneous cervical cordotomy is that some weakness may develop on the ipsilateral side. Normally there is always some added weakness in the first three postoperative days, presumably due to oedema of the spinal cord. This settles and the patient recovers that power he had at the end of the cordotomy. Of patients who have a unilateral percutaneous cervical cordotomy carried out with the precautions mentioned, 90 per cent do not have sufficient weakness to prevent them walking; 40 per cent appreciate that the ipsilateral leg is weak, with half of these (20 per cent) having to be careful when they walk up or down stairs or turn round on the flat. The remaining 10 per cent of patients will require the use of a walking aid or knee brace because of weakness of the leg, but three-quarters of them will not need these supports beyond the first month. It must be remembered that in the 2·5 per cent of patients who still require a walking aid beyond one month will be those who have been bed-ridden for some considerably time or who also had mild paresis previously.

It must be emphasized once again that this is an excellent method for the relief of pain in cancer in a patient who has an expectation of life of up to 2 years, especially if the pain is confined to one side of the body. If pain is present on both sides of the body then a bilateral cordotomy or a combination of cordotomy, lateral and anterior, or a cordotomy plus intrathecal phenol may be necessary. Over 80 per cent of patients obtain total relief of unilateral pain with the unilateral PCC. Most patients who have a percutaneous cervical cordotomy will be ambulant one or two days postoperatively. A few will be confined to bed for longer periods because of an associated headache.

References

Crue, B. L. Jr, Todd, E. M., Carregal, E. J. A., Wright, W. H. and Maline, D. B. (1970). Posterior approach for high cervical radiofrequency stereotactic cordotomy. *Pain and Suffering—selected aspects*, Chapter 5. Ed. by B. L. Crue, Jr. Thomas, Springfield, Illinois.

Ganz, E. and Mullan, S. (1977). Percutaneous cordotomy. *Persistent Pain*, Vol. 1, p. 31. Ed. by S. Lipton. Academic Press, London and New York.

Lin, P. M., Gildenberg, P. L. and Polakoff, P. P. (1966). An anterior approach to percutaneous lower cervical cordotomy. *Journal of Neurosurgery* **25**, 553.

Lipton, S. (1968). Percutaneous electrical cordotomy in relief of intractable pain. *British Medical Journal* **2**, 210.

Lipton, S., Dervin, E. and Heywood, O. B. (1974). A stereotactic approach to the anterior percutaneous electrical cordotomy. In: *Advances in Neurology*, Vol. 4, p. 689. Ed. by J. J. Bonica. Raven Press, New York.

Mullan, S. and Hosobuchi, Y. (1968). Respiratory hazards of high cervical percutaneous cordotomy. *Journal of Neurosurgery* **22**, 291.

Mullan, S., Harper, P. V., Hekmatapanah, J., Torres, H. and Dobbin, G. (1963). Percutaneous interruption of spinal pain tracts by means of a strontium 90 needle. *Journal of Neurosurgery* **20**, 931.

Mullan, S., Mallis, M., Karasick, J., Vailati, G. and Beckman, F. (1965). A reappraisal of the unipolar anodal electrolytic lesion. *Journal of Neurosurgery* **22**, 531.

Rosomoff, H. L. (1969). Bilateral percutaneous cervical radiofrequency cordotomy. *Journal of Neurosurgery* **31**, 41.

Rosomoff, H. L., Carroll, F., Brown, J. and Sheptak, P. (1965). Percutaneous radiofrequency cervical cordotomy technique. *Journal of Neurosurgery* **23**, 639.

Spiller, W. G. and Martin, E. (1912). The treatment of persistent pain of organic origin in the lower part of the body by division of the antero-lateral column of the spinal cord. *Journal of the American Medical Association* **58**, 1489.

15
Pituitary injection of alcohol

It has long been known that occasionally a malignant condition stops grow-ing, and very occasionally regresses completely. This occurs particularly in hormone-dependent tumours of the breast and prostate, and surgical male or female castration, adrenalectomy and, finally, pituitary ablation have been used to treat these conditions (Leading article, 1969; Hayward *et al.*, 1970).

Since 1968 Moricca has advocated destruction of the pituitary gland with alcohol for the relief of pain in patients with any form of carcinoma and also for those patients who have hormone-dependent tumours (Moricca, 1974, 1976, 1977; Tindall *et al.*, 1977). The technique is simple to carry out using an image intensifier with television attachment to control the position of the needles. A transnasal, trans-sphenoidal approach is made with a 15 gauge trocar and cannula 15 cm long. The sphenoid sinus lies behind the pos-terior nasal fossa, there being a stoma on each side; above the sphenoid sinus and somewhat posteriorly, lies the pituitary fossa separated from the sphenoid sinus by thin bone. The trocar and cannula is inserted through the nose into the sphenoid sinus and on through the bone at the base of the pitui-tary fossa into or near the pituitary gland (Fig. 15.1). The trocar is aimed about 2 mm inferior to the posterior clinoid processes so that, if it penetrates too deeply, it impinges on bone and does not go deeper.

The procedure is carried out under either local or general anaesthesia, but general anaesthesia is preferable because alcohol spilling over into the middle fossa produces severe headache. The cannula must be kept in the midline, otherwise it enters the cavernous sinus and venous or arterial haemorrhage results. Radio-opaque material is injected into the pituitary fossa and can be seen on the lateral x-ray film. This ensures that the cannula is in the correct position. A total of not more than 1·0 ml dehydrated alcohol (100 per cent) is injected in divided doses, with the pupillary light reflex and the size of the pupils being monitored between each increment. The alcohol spreads into the cerebrospinal fluid, past the stalk of the pituitary gland and, because it is hypobaric and the patient lies in the dorsal position, it will float past the optic nerve and the optic chiasma.

When the procedure is being carried out for a hormone-dependent tumour then, if the patient's condition is good enough, three pituitary injections are

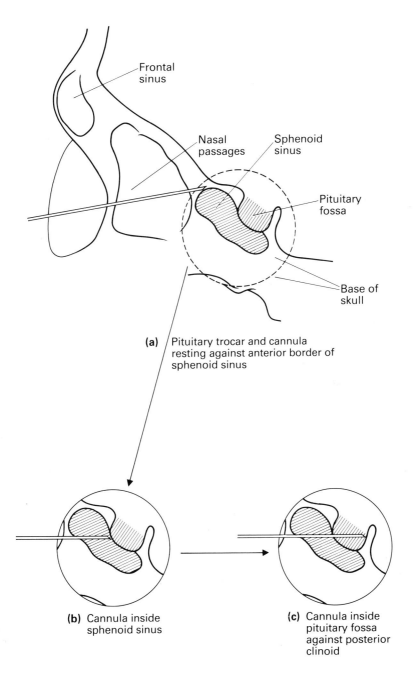

(a) Pituitary trocar and cannula
resting against anterior border of
sphenoid sinus

(b) Cannula inside
sphenoid sinus

(c) Cannula inside
pituitary fossa
against posterior
clinoid

Fig. 15.1   Insertion of pituitary cannula

carried out within three weeks; if pain is the major presenting symptom, the number of injections depends on the result after the initial pituitary injection of alcohol. If pain is relieved completely, no further injections are carried out until it recurs. If the pain is partially relieved or is completely relieved and then returns, a further pituitary injection is carried out after one week and, if further improvement is achieved, a third injection is carried out one week later. If pain is relieved completely after the second injection no further injections are performed. However, if after two pituitary injections there has been no relief at all the method is abandoned as unsuitable.

The pituitary injection of alcohol appears to be effective in relieving pain in tumours which are not usually considered to be hormone-dependent. The type of tumour does not seem to be critical although there is a preponderance of patients with carcinoma of the breast and prostate in our results. Sometimes when iophendylate is injected into the pituitary fossa it is seen to pass along the stalk, round the floor of the third ventricle, eventually breaking through into the cavity of the third ventricle. It is reasonable to assume that the alcohol also spreads along this pathway and the possibility of pain relief occurring through direct hypothalamic injury has to be considered. This is supported by the work of Sano (1973), who obtained relief of pain in 50 per cent of his patients after destroying the posterior hypothalamus by a stereotactic approach. In a cadaver study after standard transnasal, transsphenoidal puncture of the pituitary fossa, a mixture of Indian ink and iophendylate (Myodil) was injected (Miles and Lipton, 1976); in 5 out of 13 cases the contrast spread into the third ventricle and on 2 occasions air also passed into the third ventricle. In 3 cases contrast passed into the venous system, the spread occurring either into the basal veins and into the great cerebral vein or through the petrosal sinus to the transverse sinus. In all except 1 case, Indian ink was seen in the pituitary gland itself and in every case the pituitary stalk contained dye, as did the blood vessels, particularly the large peripheral portal vessels and the walls of these vessels. In all 13 cases dye was seen in sections of the hypothalamus. It thus appears that fluid injected into the pituitary gland spreads rapidly from this site and that it spreads mainly in the lumen of blood vessels although rupture through the walls also occurs.

Practically, this technique is extremely useful because it deals with bilateral cancer pain from a widespread primary tumour or from secondary tumours, and does not have to be confined to spinal segments. It will also relieve pain in the head and neck (Lipton et al., 1978). The percentage relief of pain is not as great as in the percutaneous cervical cordotomy, being of the order of 70 per cent, while 30 per cent are unaffected. Of those patients who obtain pain relief, 40 per cent are completely relieved of pain for a period of time while 30 per cent obtain partial relief. Of the 40 per cent of patients who have complete relief, half of them (20 per cent) have relief of pain for more than four months. When pain recurs the injection is repeated.

As might be expected, complications can result from the alcohol spreading on to the optic nerves and chiasma, and the nearby cranial nerves. In all our 165 pituitary injections there were no permanent deficits. Mortality was of the order of 5 per cent, and most (but not all) patients had a diabetes insipidus of mild degree for up to two weeks, although in a few patients it persisted for six weeks. The diabetes insipidus could be easily controlled by the use of desmopressin (DDAVP) oily nasal drops three or four times per day. In our series the pain relief has been of great value; we have had no obvious cases of regression of tumour although Moricca in his much larger series has incontrovertible evidence that this can occur.

References

Hayward, J. L., Atkins, H. J. B., Falconer, M. A., MacLean, K. S., Salmon, L. F. W., Schurr, P. H. and Shaheen, C. H. (1970). Clinical trials comparing transfrontal hypophysectomy with adrenalectomy and with transethmoidal hypophysectomy. In: *The Clinical Management of Advanced Breast Cancer*. Ed. by C. A. F. Joslin and E. N. Gleave. Alpha Omega Alpha, Cardiff.

Leading article (1969). Treatment of advanced breast cancer. *British Medical Journal* **1**, 265.

Lipton, S., Miles, J. B., Williams, N., Bark-Jones, N. (1978). Pituitary injection of alcohol for widespread cancer pain. *Pain* **5**, 73–82.

Miles, J. and Lipton, S. (1976). The mode of action by which pituitary alcohol injection relieves pain. In: *Advances in Pain Research and Therapy*, Vol. 1, p. 867. Ed. by J. J. Bonica and D. Albe-Fessard. Raven Press, New York.

Moricca, G. (1968). *Progress in Anaesthesiology*. Proceedings of the Fourth World Congress of Anaesthesiologists, p. 266. Excerpta Medica, Amsterdam.

Moricca, G. (1974). Chemical hypophysectomy for cancer pain. *Advances in Neurology*, Vol. 4, p. 707. Ed. by J. J. Bonica. Raven Press, New York.

Moricca, G. (1976). Neuroadenolysis (chemical hypophysectomy) for diffuse unbearable cancer pain. In: *Advances in Pain Research and Therapy*, Vol. 1, p. 863. Ed. by J. J. Bonica and D. Albe-Fessard. Raven Press, New York.

Moricca, G. (1977). Pituitary neuroadenylysis in the treatment of intractable pain from cancer. In: *Persistent Pain*, Vol. 1, p. 149. Ed. by S. Lipton. Academic Press, London and New York.

Sano, K. (1973). Presented to Symposium Sur la Doleur, September 24, Paris.

Tindall, C. T., Nixon, D. W., Christy, J. H. *et al* (1977). Pain relief in metastatic cancer other than breast and prostate gland following transsphenoidal hypophysectomy. *Journal of Neurosurgery* **47**, 659.

16
The facet joint

Most pain in the back or neck which does not arise from the soft tissues, arises from a prolapsed intervertebral disc or from osteophytes pressing on the nerve root and this is discussed in Chapter 9. However, it is possible that some of this pain arises at the posterior facet joints (intervertebral or zygoapophyseal). The territory of the posterior primary rami of the spinal nerves covers an area from the vertex to the coccyx, extending laterally to the border of the trapezius, the acromion, the scapula, on to the trochanter and finally to the coccyx (Bradley, 1974).

The posterior primary ramus divides into a lateral and a medial branch. Although there are differences at different spinal levels, essentially the medial branch supplies an area from the midline to the line of the posterior vertebral joints. It supplies the lower portion of the joint capsule at its level of exit and then passes downwards, supplying the upper portion of the capsule of the facet joint below.

Thus, for any single facet joint to be rendered insensitive, two posterior primary rami have to be blocked: the one above and the one at its own level. This is quite easily carried out by two local injections. One at the base of the superior articular facet of the facet joint which is to be blocked, and another at the same position at the facet joint immediately below. In the lumbar region the descending branch grooves the bone between the transverse process and the inferior facet joint.

To block these nerves in the lumbar region the patient lies prone and, by the use of an image intensifier, the facet joints are identified. The skin is marked at the point of injection above each superior facet joint along the line of joints to be injected. Insertion of the 5-cm 20 gauge needle is made without difficulty; when it touches bone, the position is checked with the image intensifier. Bupivacaine (3 ml of 0·5 per cent) with 1 in 200 000 adrenaline will produce 6–8 hours' anaesthesia of the joints in the lumbar region. This will provide a good diagnostic test for pain relief. Sometimes during the injection of a particular facet joint, pain will be referred to the back or sacral region and, occasionally, to the buttock or upper posterior thigh. On rare occasions, pain is referred from a facet joint on one side of the body to the opposite side.

To block the cervical facets, the image intensifier is set at an angle of about 45 degrees so that a view is obtained down the vertebral foramen. The needle is inserted until it appears on the x-ray immediately posterior to the foramen, resting against bone. In this position it is well away from the intervertebral nerve.

When diagnostic tests are positive (i.e. pain relief occurs and is repeatable) these nerves can be destroyed by a radiofrequency current heat coagulation (Mehta and Sluijter, 1977). It is best to keep the amount of heat produced to a reasonable level; therefore, the temperature of the coagulating probe is not allowed to rise above 80° C for more than 40 seconds.

References

Bradley, K. C. (1974). The anatomy of backache. *Australian and New Zealand Journal of Surgery* **44**, 227–232.
Mehta, M. and Sluijter, M. E. (1977). Paper read at the Boerhaave course 'Anaesthetists and Pain Relief'. May 1977, Leiden, Netherlands.

Further reading

Oudenhoven, R. C. (1974). Articular rhizotomy. *Surgical Neurology* **2**, 257–258.
Pedersen, H. E., Blunck, C. F. J. and Gardner, E. (1956). The anatomy of lumbosacral posterior rami and meningeal branches of spinal nerves (sinu-vertebral nerves). *Journal of Bone and Joint Surgery* **38A**, 377–391.
Rees, W. E. S. (1971). Multiple bilateral subcutaneous rhizolysis of segmental nerves in the treatment of the intervertebral disc syndrome. *Annals of General Practice* **16**, 126–127.
Shealy, C. N. (1974). The role of the spinal facets in back and sciatic pain. *Headache* **4**, 101–104.
Toakley, J. G. (1973). Subcutaneous lumbar 'rhizolysis'—an assessment of 200 cases. *Medical Journal of Australia* **2**, 490–492.

17
Nerve blocks

The technique of nerve blocking has been improved by a number of features.

The introduction of the amide local anaesthetics which diffuse widely in the body tissues has allowed successful blocks to be achieved despite less accurate positioning of the needle. On occasion, the older esters such as procaine are valuable when a very limited block is required for diagnostic purpose. For instance, procaine may be useful when a permanent trigeminal ganglion block is to be made and the extent of the block and the possibility of third nerve palsies are tested.

The use of the semi-portable image intensifier has simplified many techniques by allowing visualization of the bony structures and the needle. The image intensifier is a small combined unit which involves an x-ray machine linked to television equipment so that an immediate view of the tissues in the x-ray beam is seen on the television screen. This is invaluable in carrying out nerve blocks, or plexus blocks, where positioning of the needle is difficult but is rendered relatively easy by the use of rapid x-ray views. The head of the image intensifier swings through 90 degrees so that anteroposterior or lateral views can be obtained. The latest models have memory facilities.

The nerve stimulator, or block aid monitor which is connected to a metal needle, insulated throughout its length except for a few millimetres at the tip, is an aid to accurate localization of the needle. Stimulation of this needle with a suitable current at 2 Hz gives motor stimulation while stimulation at 50 or 100 Hz tends to give sensory stimulation. This apparatus can be used when the nerve is buried or situated in an inaccessible place. The proximity of the needle tip to the nerve can be estimated from the amount of current necessary to produce stimulation. When the stimulation is minimal, the nerve and the needle tip are very close indeed.

When an electric current is passed through a needle the electric flux is maximal at the tip; therefore, provided the current is not too high, the stimulation along the length of the needle is relatively small while the tip is active and will stimulate nerves in a selective fashion but not, of course, as effectively as when they are insulated.

Various anaesthetic drugs are available. Common ones are benzocaine, procaine (Novocain) and chloroprocaine (Nesacaine). Chloroprocaine is the least toxic of these and they are all esters of para-aminobenzoic acid. This group of local anaesthetics diffuses much less easily than the larger group of local anaesthetic drugs which are amines. The amines include such well known anaesthetic substances as lignocaine (Xylocaine), prilocaine (Citanest), etidocaine (Duranest) and bupivacaine (Marcain). The last two have the longest effect and are the least toxic. Bupivacaine 0·5 per cent with 1 in 200 000 adrenaline will give anaesthesia for up to ten hours.

One difference between the esters and the amide groups of local anaesthetic agents has been mentioned; another is that the esters are hydrolysed by plasma cholinesterase, which means that patients with a deficiency of plasma cholinesterase do not hydrolyse these drugs at the usual rate and thus there is a reduced tolerance. Further, if a general anaesthetic is given to cover the injection and suxamethonium chloride (Anectine) is included in the general anaesthetic, a prolonged neuromuscular block may occur, with an added risk of toxicity when the local anaesthetic used is an ester. Thus, under these circumstances it is best to use an amide local anaesthetic agent because these are metabolized mainly by microsomal enzymes in the liver. As a corollary, if the patient has liver disease, then amide drugs may need to be reduced in quantity or an ester anaesthetic agent may be preferred.

The toxic effects and duration of an anaesthetic block are a function of the total dose of the local anaesthetic used. There are as many toxic effects produced when equivalent doses are used in a dilute solution as in a concentrated solution. Naturally, if injection is made into a blood vessel or a vascular portion of the body then toxic effects are more likely. Thus, overall toxic effects depend on the dosage, the pharmacological structure of the drug, the technique of injection and the position of the injection.

When a long-lasting block is required, different drugs are used; the two substances commonly used are alcohol and phenol. In small quantities, 100 per cent alcohol may be injected peripherally but, as this may produce neuritis, it tends to be employed only under special circumstances. Alcohol is used for intrathecal nerve blocks, particularly in the difficult mid-thoracic position. In the cerebrospinal fluid it is a hypobaric substance and will float to the uppermost portion of the c.s.f. Thus, if the nerve which is to be affected is positioned in such a way that it is at the highest portion of the spinal theca, then alcohol injected at a lower level will float up to that point and affect the required nerve.

The other common substance is phenol, and various concentrations are used. The strongest concentration that can be produced approaches 8 per cent. However, in most cases, concentrations of 6 per cent are used for injections in tissues and either 1 in 20 phenol in glycerine or 1 in 15 phenol in glycerine are used for intrathecal injections. Phenol in glycerine is a hyperbaric solution and will flow to the lowermost part of the spinal theca. Thus, when used intrathecally the nerve to be affected is placed at the most dependent part of the spinal theca. However, one important difference between 100 per cent alcohol and phenol in glycerine is in the viscosity of the substance. Phenol in glycerine is very viscous and therefore will move slowly from one portion of the spinal theca to another whilst hypobaric alcohol will flow readily.

By using in succession 2 per cent benzocaine in arachis oil, followed by twice the quantity of 6 per cent urethane injected down the same needle without any movement of the needle, an effective long-acting block is achieved. Mixing occurs in the tissues. This is useful for easily accessible nerves such as subcostal blocks for secondary carcinoma in a rib.

Autonomic blocks

There are three blocks of the autonomic nervous system which are used frequently: (1) the stellate ganglion block, (2) the lumbar sympathetic block and (3) the coeliac plexus block.

1. Stellate ganglion

This ganglion is formed by the inferior cervical ganglion and the first thoracic ganglion. When these are two separate structures, the inferior cervical ganglion lies in front of the seventh cervical transverse process and the first thoracic ganglion lies in front of the neck of the first rib. Usually, the stellate ganglion is a single structure lying along the neck of the first rib and spreading upwards into the space above. The technique of blocking this ganglion depends on depositing anaesthetic solution anterior to the neck of the first rib. Alternatively, the injection can be made below, and anterior to, the transverse process of the seventh cervical vertebra.

The stellate ganglion is injected direct only if it is desired to destroy the ganglion by means of alcohol or phenol. Normally, a much simpler technique is used for diagnostic blocks, as the stellate ganglion forms part of the sympathetic trunk which, in the cervical region, lies behind the carotid sheath on the fascia covering the muscles. A little further posterior are the transverse processes of the cervical vertebrae. Below and in front is the pleura.

Thus, if a needle is placed anterior to a transverse process of mid or lower cervical vertebra so that it first touches bone and is then withdrawn slightly, its tip should then be anterior to the fascia covering the muscles. An injection of 10 ml of 1 per cent lignocaine will diffuse downwards on the fascia, especially if the patient is half reclining, to produce a stellate ganglion block. When the needle tip is in the correct position the injection is very simple and can be made without much pressure.

2. Lumbar sympathetic chain

In the lumbar region the sympathetic chain lies on the anterolateral surface of the lumbar vertebrae. The twelfth thoracic and first lumbar ganglia are frequently joined together. Sometimes some of the other ganglia fuse so that only three or four lumbar ganglia are present. There is no constant position for these ganglia, and their position varies from side to side. The most constant ganglion is that found in relation to the body of the second lumbar vertebra, and when a one needle technique is used it is usually placed at this level.

The ganglia on each side lie medial to the origin of the psoas muscle against the anterolateral portion of the vertebral body. Anterior on the right side is the inferior vena cava and on the left side is the aorta. They are covered by retroperitoneal fascia and this produces a fascial compartment limited by the vertebral column, psoas sheath and retroperitoneal fascia. Because this contains the lumbar sympathetic chain, anaesthetic solutions placed in this compartment can travel up and down the chain and will have a wide effect.

One injection technique

A skin weal is made lateral to the spinous process to the second lumbar verte-bra and a needle inserted through it until it touches the transverse process. This distance is approximately 5 cm, and the distance to the lumbar chain is twice that. The depth marker can be placed 5 cm from the skin when the tip is against the transverse process; the needle is then withdrawn and reinserted so that it passes by the side of the transverse process and touches the lateral edge of the vertebra. The needle is inserted to the depth marker and, in this position, the tip of the needle will be very close to the sympathetic chain. The resistance to injection of the fascial compartment is very low.

Before a surgical lumbar sympathectomy is carried out to improve a de-ficient circulation in the lower limb, a diagnostic block of the lumbar sym-pathetic chain is often performed and the rise in limb temperature observed with a skin thermometer. It is essential that the block be complete and there-fore a similar technique to the one mentioned above is used but with three needles inserted at L2, L3, and L4.

This block, as in the corresponding stellate ganglion block for the upper limb, is useful for improving the vascular supply to the limb and in causalgia and other reflex sympathetic dystrophies.

The use of the lumbar sympathetic block in intermittent claudication is usually of only temporary benefit, as the underlying vascular condition is progressive; with a fixed blood volume flowing into the limb, the sympathetic blockade may merely rearrange the circulation between skin and muscle com-ponents.

3. Coeliac plexus

The coeliac plexus is a large pre-vertebral plexus spreading over a wide area from the middle of the twelfth thoracic vertebra above, to the middle of the second lumbar vertebra below. It lies between the two adrenal glands later-ally while behind it is the aorta lying between the crura of the diaphragm, and to the right and anteriorly is the inferior vena cava.

The plexus is surrounded by loose areolar tissue and thus any injection designed to affect this plexus is made about 1 cm anterior to the anterior border of the first lumbar vertebra. Here it is very close to the large vessels and care must be taken not to inject anaesthetic solution directly into them; if the needle does penetrate a major vessel, it is withdrawn until aspiration of blood is negative and then cautiously re-advanced, injecting saline ahead of the needle. In this way, vessels can be pushed out of the way but the later injection of anaesthetic solution tends to be diluted. Anaesthesia of this plexus produces vasodilatation of the lower half of the body and the lower limbs with hypotension of a marked degree, especially in the older patient. This block also interrupts the afferent fibres from the upper abdominal viscera carrying pain, so that the coeliac plexus block is particularly useful for relieving the pain of inoperable cancer of the upper abdominal organs. It is also useful in treating the pain of chronic pancreatitis.

Bridenbaugh's technique (Bridenbaugh, Moore and Campbell, 1964) is recommended for blocking this structure. The needle is inserted about 5 cm from the midline and is directed anterior to the twelfth thoracic vertebra. It is directed parallel to the twelfth rib and below it. If it goes above the twelfth rib (i.e. cephalad) it may enter the pleura. The transverse process of the first lumbar vertebra has to be negotiated just as in a lumbar sympathetic block, and a long (15 cm) needle of 20 gauge or more should be used. A smaller gauge needle makes the injection extremely difficult because of the pressure needed to inject viscous fluids; also, when an image intensifier is used, a 22 gauge needle cannot be easily seen in thick-bodied patients.

Lignocaine (15 ml of 1 per cent) can be injected on each side as a diagnostic block but if a permanent block is required then 25 ml of 50 per cent alcohol are injected on each side. It is not usual to proceed with the permanent block immediately after the diagnostic block because of the dilution of the alcohol which results.

When a permanent coeliac plexus block is made in an elderly person it may last a considerable time and the ensuing hypotension must be monitored. The blood pressure is taken with the patient lying flat, and taken again after he has been sitting up for a few minutes. Then it is taken after sitting on the edge of the bed with the feet hanging over the edge and eventually standing up. Sometimes the hypotension is so profound that the foot of the bed has to be elevated with the patient lying flat.

Simple measures will raise the blood pressure; for example, bilateral thigh-length elastic stockings, an abdominal binder and, if necessary, a long-acting vasopressor such as ephedrine. Gradually over a period of a month these measures can be discontinued, one by one, until the patient can manage without them. The danger of hypotension must not be under-estimated, otherwise these patients will faint, fall and damage themselves, or develop cerebral hypoxia.

Somatic nerve blocks

A number of somatic nerve blocks are in general use and a short description of the principles and details underlying the techniques are given here. In addition, the few recent innovations into nerve blocking are also mentioned.

Blocks of the trigeminal nerve and its branches are of supreme importance because of their value in the treatment of trigeminal neuralgia.

Trigeminal nerve

This nerve can be blocked peripherally or centrally, and at the periphery these are performed where the branches are vulnerable as they leave the skull or enter the face. Thus, the supraorbital block, the infraorbital block and the mental block are carried out relatively easily and, of these, the first two are important.

Supraorbital nerve

This nerve normally divides into two branches after it crosses the edge of the orbit, forming a medial and lateral branch, and thus it can be felt in or near the superior orbital notch. Sometimes the supraorbital nerve divides into its two branches before it reaches the edge of the orbit; in this case the lateral branch is the larger. The smaller supratrochlear nerve lies medial to the supraorbital nerve at the superior medial angle of the orbit. The supraorbital nerve is blocked at, or near, the supraorbital notch and can be injected direct whilst the supratrochlear nerve is injected at the root of the nose between the upper and medial borders of the orbit. For a diagnostic block the anaesthetic solution can easily be deposited near the nerve. If alcohol is to be used then parasthesiae must be obtained and direct injection made into the nerve (or nerves).

Infraorbital nerve

This is the continuation of the maxillary division and emerges on the maxilla through the infraorbital foramen. The nerve can be blocked through the mucosa of the mouth. This is the approach normally used by dental surgeons, but most doctors use the extraoral route in which a small, 23-gauge 2·5-cm needle is inserted into the infraorbital canal. The stoma of the infraorbital canal lies below the inferior orbital ridge, about 3 cm from the midline, and can sometimes be palpated through the skin. The direction into the canal is upwards and outwards but when the foramen is not entered easily a search pattern to find it has to be made over the small area of bone where it normally lies. The patient will often mention paraesthesiae when the tip of the needle is near the foramen and, as the nerve spreads radially, paraesthesiae to the lower lid, nose, or lip indicate the direction of the foramen.

    Injections into the infraorbital canal are small—in volume not more than 1·0 ml—and it must be remembered that they may spread along the foramen into the orbit. Neurolytic agents must be injected slowly in increments and care taken to check for developing diplopia.

Inferior dental nerve

A very useful and commonly required block is the inferior dental nerve block. This enters the bone of the lower jaw through the mandibular foramen on the inner aspect of the ramus of the mandible, midway between the anterior and posterior borders and about 1 cm above the occlusal surface of the last molar tooth. A small quantity of anaesthetic solution deposited close to this foramen will anaesthetize the teeth of one side of the lower jaw and the mental region. The lingual nerve also is very close to this point and if some solution diffuses downwards, anaesthesia of the anterior two-thirds of the tongue will result as well. This is a common occurrence when an inferior dental block is carried out for dentistry. It must thus be remembered that the teeth alone are anaesthetized and not the mucous membrane round them, which needs to be anaesthetized separately.

There are two other useful blocks made on peripheral nerves: the maxillary and mandibular nerves. The motor branch of the trigeminal nerve joins the mandibular branch in the canal of the foramen ovale, and at about 1 cm below the skull the mandibular nerve splits into its various branches. These are, from before backwards, the buccal nerve, the lingual nerve and the inferior alveolar nerve. Therefore, when a lateral approach is made to this nerve, some idea of the position of the main branch can be obtained from the paraesthesiae produced.

Mandibular nerve

The technique of the lateral approach to the mandibular nerve is based on the fact that it is 4·5–5·0 cm medial to the midpoint of the zygoma. An approach from below the midpoint of the zygoma will, first of all, touch the lateral pterygoid plate at about 4 cm depth; the needle is worked posteriorly until it slips past the pterygoid plate to a depth of a further 1 cm, where it should be very close to the foramen ovale and, therefore, the mandibular nerve. If the needle is allowed to go too far posteriorly, then pain in the ear is obtained from the eustachian tube. Alcohol must not be injected into the eustachian tube, otherwise pain and vertigo for some days will result. A preliminary injection of local anaesthetic should be made in this region and if the needle is in the eustachian tube the patient will report fluid in the pharynx. When the needle is close to the nerve, dense analgesia with small volumes of solution develops rapidly. The Block-aid monitor is valuable for these blocks, (Greenblatt and Denson, 1962).

Maxillary nerve

The approach to this nerve is similar to that for the mandibular nerve. A needle is inserted below the midpoint of the zygomatic arch perpendicular to the skin until it touches the lateral pterygoid plate. The depth marker is moved 1 cm from the skin, the needle is withdrawn and re-inserted, aiming 1 cm anterior and 1 cm above the first point of contact, which allows it to enter the pterygopalatine fossa close to the maxillary nerve. It is important in this block to make sure that the needle is not inserted too deep. Medially and above the pterygopalatine fossa lies the infraorbital fissure which leads into the orbit. The injection of a large volume can produce a temporary proptosis and, similarly, a haemorrhage from the maxillary artery produces the same result with a haematoma.

Gasserian ganglion

The gasserian ganglion can be reached thriough the foramen ovale from the lateral approach, as this foramen points downwards and outwards. An alternative approach is through the same foramen from a point about 3 cm lateral to the corner of the mouth. This is the anterolateral technique of Härtel, which makes use of the fact that the foramen ovale is a relatively large foramen through which the mandibular nerve exits from the skull. This foramen is in constant position about 4·5 cm medial to the tubercle of the zygoma and about 7 cm posterior to the pupil. Anterior to the foramen ovale is the infratemporal surface of the greater wing of the sphenoid which is quite smooth—and this can be appreciated as smooth when the injection needle touches it. Posterior to the foramen ovale is the petrous portion of the temporal bone which is rough, and this also can be appreciated. In this way, with experience, it is possible to know whether the needle tip is anterior or posterior to the foramen without the use of check x-rays. However, the use of x-rays does simplify and shorten the procedure and saves the patient much trauma. Nowadays, x-ray facilities should always be used if they are available.

The direction the injection needle must take to pass through the foramen ovale is aligned by the use of surface markings. A line is drawn laterally from the corner of the mouth and a mark is made on it, at the level of the second molar tooth or at a point 3 cm posterior to the corner of the mouth, or a line is dropped from the lateral edge of the bony orbit on to it. All these three methods give approximately the same point. A line is drawn along the inferior border of the zygoma and the midpoint of the zygomatic arch marked. One line is then drawn from the point 3 cm lateral to the corner of the mouth to the mid-zygomatic point and another line to the pupil with the patient staring straight ahead. The technique is to insert a needle through the point lateral to the mouth, keeping to the two directions marked. When the needle touches bone at approximately 5 cm deep, the skin marker is then set 1·5 cm from the skin. The needle tip should impinge on the smooth bone anterior to the foramen ovale. The needle is then withdrawn and redirected about 1 cm posteriorly; it should enter the foramen ovale when the skin marker is still about 1 cm from the skin. At this depth paraesthesiae may be obtained from the mandibular nerve but this does not always occur. When the skin marker is flush with the skin, the tip of the needle has passed through the foramen ovale and lies in or near the gasserian ganglion. If the needle is inserted a further 1 cm, its tip will lie beyond Meckel's cave in cerebrospinal fluid and very close to, or in, the fasciculi of the trigeminal nerve between the pons and the posterior surface of the gasserian ganglion.

Injections of local anaesthetic agents at any of these levels will produce corresponding anaesthesia and, if local anaesthetic spills over on to adjacent cranial nerves, ocular palsy and diplopia will result. The older technique of blocking the trigeminal nerve involved injecting a small quantity of local anaesthetic solution into the gasserian ganglion to see what divisions were affected and then using fractional doses of neurolytic agents to obtain the required analgesia. During this procedure, monitoring of diplopia and pupillary size was carried out.

The modern technique is to use a needle electrode with a bared tip of 0·5 cm (sometimes 1·0 cm) and to place this tip amongst the retrogasserian fasciculi (Sweet and Wepsic, 1974). Stimulation by a suitable stimulating electric current will produce sensation in one or more divisions of the trigeminal nerve. By moving the needle electrode a few millimetres in or out, stimulation of the desired division or divisions can be obtained and a radiofrequency current heat coagulation of these retrogasserian fibres can be carried out in a controlled fashion. In this way analgesia gradually develops and deepens and, if required, anaesthesia can be obtained. Usually, analgesia only is desired, as it is believed that a little residual sensation in the face prevents the development of anaesthesia dolorosa. (In this condition the patient has an anaesthetic, yet painful face.)

The nearer the needle electrode is inserted to the corner of the mouth, the more likely it is to affect the third division. The further away from the corner of the mouth, the more medial is its insertion through the foramen ovale and the more likely it is to affect first division fibres. This is an important practical point because affecting the first division will obtund the corneal reflex and render the patient liable to infection and damage to the eye.

Brachial plexus block

The brachial plexus is formed by the anterior primary rami of the fifth, sixth, seventh and eighth cervical nerves and the first thoracic nerve; occasionally, C4 and T2 are included. The various portions of the brachial plexus unite and separate in a complicated fashion, and between the anterior and middle scalene muscles the three trunks are formed. These three trunks cross the upper border of the first rib, lateral to the subclavian artery and lie between the insertion of the middle scalene muscle posteriorly and the anterior scalene muscle anteriorly. The brachial plexus can be blocked easily at the point where it crosses the first rib. The essentials of the technique are that a needle is placed in contact with the first rib lateral to the subclavian artery; 10 ml of solution is deposited at this point after aspiration; if a sensory block only is required, 1 or 1·5 per cent lignocaine is used, while 2 per cent lignocaine produces a motor block.

There is a fascial compartment extending from the anterior and middle scalene muscles laterally and in this lies the brachial plexus and the subclavian artery. If local anaesthetic solution is deposited in this, the whole of the brachial plexus can be anaesthetized.

In the axillary approach method the axillary artery is palpated with the arm abducted to 90 degrees and the needle is inserted towards and slightly above the artery. At this point the plexus lies superficially around the artery and a deep injection causes the block to fail. Gentleness is important during the insertion of the needle because a haematoma forming within the fascial sheath will prevent effective anaesthesia.

After placing the needle, a vibration transmitted from the needle to the artery will show that it lies within the fascial compartment; after aspiration, about 20 ml of 1·5 or 2 per cent lignocaine is injected. The fascial compartment extends along the artery and it is best to place a tourniquet below the injection point to block it off so that the injected solution must spread upwards.

The advantage of the axillary approach is that there is no danger of a pneumothorax—a problem ever present with the supraclavicular approach.

Somatic spinal nerve block

One of the most convenient places to block a spinal nerve is as it leaves the spinal foramen, and the methods of doing this vary at different levels. It must be remembered that in the pain relief clinic it is not necessary to block a wide area to resolve the problem of which particular nerves are transmitting painful stimuli.

There are eight pairs of cervical nerves, the first emerging above the first vertebra, and the eighth below the seventh vertebra. The posterior primary rami divide into medial sensory and lateral motor branches, with the medial branches supplying the skin of the posterior part of the neck and the occipital scalp. The cervical second and third medial branches form the greater occipital nerve and the third occipital nerve. The anterior primary divisions of the upper four cervical nerves form the cervical plexus and the lower four go to form the brachial plexus. Lateral to the foramina, the nerve and primary divisions lie posterior to the vertebral artery in a groove in the transverse process. These transverse processes have an anterior and posterior tubercle of which the posterior tubercle is the larger, and it is much easier to approach the nerve laterally than posteriorly. When making an injection in this region it is best to direct the injecting needle from above downwards on to a transverse process, as it is much more difficult to enter the spinal theca with this approach.

Cervical plexus block

A deep cervical plexus block is performed from the lateral approach unless there is tumour tissue or an abscess present in this direction. A line is drawn from the mastoid process to the prominent sixth transverse process (Chassaignac's). The second transverse process is 1·5 cm inferior to the mastoid process on this line, with the other transverse processes 1·5 cm below the one above. A needle is inserted through the skin to the transverse process which it meets at a depth of about 3 cm, and no injection is made until bone is contacted. When all three needles are in the correct positions (C2, C3, C4), they will be in a line.

C2 nerve block

This block is often made with lignocaine for the diagnosis of pain in the occipital distribution. If it produces relief of the symptoms, it is then followed by an injection of absolute alcohol. Alcohol should not be injected unless paraesthesiae are produced. When carrying out this particular block, or any others along the bony spine, the use of an image intensifier is a great help.

Owing to the presence of the vertebral artery and other large vessels close to the cervical nerves, an aspiration test must be carried out before injection. In addition, the phrenic nerve takes its roots from C3, C4 and C5 and paralysis of the diaphragm on one side can result. Similarly, the laryngeal nerve can be affected, producing a hoarse voice, while a subarachnoid injection is possible through the intervertebral space or into a prolongation of dura around the spinal nerve. Should this occur, total spinal anaesthesia may be produced. Another possible complication is a cervical sympathetic block, which will produce a Horner's syndrome.

Greater occipital nerve block

The greater occipital nerve is blocked medial to the occipital artery which can be palpated approximately 3 cm from the midline lateral to the external occipital protruberance. This block can be extended laterally by blocking the lesser occipital nerve 2·5–3 cm lateral to the greater occipital nerve. As the third occipital nerve is medial to the greater occipital nerve, it is blocked at the same time.

Superficial cervical plexus block

All the nerves formed from the superficial cervical plexus are blocked at the posterior border of the sternomastoid muscle. The skin weal is made 2 cm or so above that point on the sternomastoid where the external jugular vein crosses it. Injections are made in three directions, the first being vertical and penetrating the deep fascia. The second is made below deep fascia and parallel to the posterior border towards the mastoid process, and the third injection is similar to the second except that it is made downwards towards the sternal head. Again, aspiration tests are important; injection of the anaesthetic solution is best made when the needle is withdrawn. A total of 15 ml of solution, at least, is used.

Dorsal and lumbar paravertebral blocks

The same technique is used for these although the anatomy is slightly different in the two regions. This is principally the result of the difference in size, as the dorsal vertebrae are not as large as the lumbar. The injection needle is inserted lateral to the spine of one of the vertebrae until it touches the transverse process. It is then withdrawn and reinserted underneath the same transverse process but medially and deeper than the initial contact so that the final position places the tip of the needle close to the nerve at the intervertebral foramen. If the nerve is touched, paraesthesiae are obtained and the needle is not inserted any further. If paraesthesiae are not obtained, the needle is advanced carefully until it touches the body of the vertebra anterior to the nerve and it is then withdrawn 1 cm. In all cases the aspiration test is carried out before the injection is made. Another precaution is to disconnect the syringe from the needle to see if there is any leak back of c.s.f.

Paravertebral dorsal block

One of the problems in this region is that imbrication of the dorsal spinous processes is great enough to place the tip of one spinous process at a lower level than its own transverse process. In most cases, the spinous process of one vertebra is on the same plane as the intervertebral foramen of the next lower vertebra but in the mid-thoracic region it will probably be even lower than this. In some patients, the spinous process in the mid-thoracic region may be in the same plane as the transverse process of the second vertebra below.

Certain landmarks are important. The most prominent cervical spine at the base of the neck is that of the C7. Also, with the arms by the side of the body the line joining the spines of the scapulae passes through the third thoracic spine. Similarly, a line joining the inferior angles of the scapulae passes through the seventh dorsal spine.

On occasion, it is easier to count upwards from the lumbar vertebrae and a line which joins the highest point of the iliac crest passes through the L4 spine or the interspace between L4 and L5. With an image intensifier it is much easier to count from the sacrum or to see the twelfth rib and count from there. It must be remembered that sometimes there is an extra lumbar vertebra, or an apparent extra lumbar vertebra, because of lumbarization of the first sacral vertebra. Similarly, there can be sacralization of the fifth lumbar vertebra.

The spinous process overlying the transverse process of the chosen nerve is marked and the needle inserted 3 cm laterally. It will touch the transverse process, and the depth marker on the needle is then set a further 2·5 cm from the skin. The needle is withdrawn and reinserted beneath the transverse process and directed medially. When more than one nerve is injected, the needles form a straight line lateral to the spinous processes and they are parallel to each other. Often, injection down one paravertebral needle will cause a flow of solution out of the others. It must be remembered that, if skin analgesia is required, at least three adjacent nerves have to be injected because of their overlapping sensory fields.

It is possible to produce a pneumothorax but if this happens it usually settles unless a tension pneomothorax develops. If a pneumothorax occurs in an outpatient, it is essential to admit him to hospital for observation. When an image intensifier is used, both anteroposterior and lateral views are useful, but lateral views cannot be used in the upper dorsal region because the spine is masked by the scapulae and the shoulder joint.

Paravertebral lumbar block

The anterior primary rami of the upper four lumbar nerves form the lumbar plexus, and part of the fifth lumbar nerve joins the anterior primary rami of the upper three sacral nerves to form the sacral plexus.

In the lumbar region the lower edge of the spinous process of a lumbar vertebra lies at the same cross-sectional level as the intervertebral foramina, and the upper border of a lumbar spinous process is at the same cross-sectional level as the transverse process of the same vertebra. Other land-marks were mentioned above in the section on dorsal paravertebral block.

The lumbar paravertebral block technique is the same as that of the dorsal except that the skin weal is raised 4 cm from the midline and the transverse process is about 5 cm deep with the depth marker set at 3 cm from the skin. It is much easier in the lumbar region to make an unwanted subarachnoid injection.

Intercostal nerve block

It is not necessary always to carry out dorsal paravertebral block, and the intercostal nerves can be anaesthetized instead. They run in the intercostal spaces below the corresponding rib and can be blocked anywhere along their length, but there are three positions where injections can be performed rela-tively easily.

The most prominent part of a rib is the posterior angle, and blocking the nerve in this position will produce a block of the complete nerve distal to this site. Even in fat patients where the posterior angle may be several centi-metres deep, it can still be palpated easily and is the most accessible portion of the rib. Alternatively, the nerve can be blocked at the posterior axillary line, which will block all the nerves distal to it, including the lateral cutaneous branch; lastly, it can be blocked at the anterior axillary line, but an injection here will not include the lateral cutaneous branch in the nerve block.

The only important feature in carrying out a subcostal block is to make sure that a pneumothorax is not produced. A fine needle only long enough to reach 1 cm past the surface of the rib is sufficient and in the average patient a standard 23-gauge 2·5 cm needle is used. A syringe should be kept attached to the needle at all times to prevent the aspiration of air into the pleural cavity.

Normally the needle is inserted direct down to the selected rib, without a skin weal, and is then withdrawn a short distance and the needle and the tissues are slid downwards until the point can be reinserted just underneath the lower edge of the rib. The tip goes no more than 0·5 cm deeper and, after aspiration, the injection is made.

Iliohypogastric and ilioinguinal nerve block

Both these nerves arise from the first lumbar nerve and a paravertebral block produces effective anaesthesia of them both. They can also be blocked at the anterior superior iliac spine, and this is the method usually adopted. The two nerves supply the skin of the inguinal region except for part of the scro-tum and adjacent thigh which are supplied by the genitofemoral nerve. This block is often used for chronic pain which develops postoperatively following incisions into the inguinal region.

The iliohypogastric nerve and the ilioinguinal nerve cannot be blocked individually; because their courses lie intramuscularly, penetrating the trans-versus abdominis near the iliac crest, a fan injection is made across the course of these nerves so that they are anaesthetized as they pass through the anaes-thetic solution.

Lateral femoral cutaneous nerve block

The lateral femoral cutaneous nerve arises from the anterior primary divisions of the L2 and L3 nerves and enters the thigh below the lateral end of the inguinal ligament about 1 cm medial to the anterior superior iliac spine. It is in this position that the nerve is usually blocked. The nerve has a large anterior branch which supplies the skin of the anterolateral portion of the thigh down to the knee, and a smaller posterior branch which supplies the skin of the lateral portion of the buttock and upper lateral thigh below the greater trochanter.

Blocking this nerve is useful in the diagnosis and treatment of meralgia paraesthetica where there are paraesthesiae, pain and numbness in the thigh. Treatment is by repeated blocks, and steroids can be added to the solution. A permanent block can be performed with a neurolytic agent but in this case paraesthesiae must be obtained before injection. The most satisfactory way of treating this condition is to section the nerve under local anaesthesia after a local anaesthetic block has confirmed the diagnosis.

Genitofemoral nerve block

The genitofemoral nerve can be blocked paravertebrally adjacent to the L1 and L2 nerves. The nerve has a long course through the psoas muscle, finally reaching the internal inguinal ring where it divides into a genital and a femoral branch. The genital branch is distributed to the skin of the scrotum, the adjacent part of the thigh and the cremaster muscle. The femoral branch supplies the skin over the femoral triangle.

Neuralgia of this nerve simulates the neuralgia produced by the ilioinguinal and iliohypogastric nerves but there are additional features, consisting of pain over the lower portion of the abdomen, the groin, the upper portion of the thigh, the scrotum or labia and the adjacent medial thigh. Male patients complain of pain in the testes. The treatment, after paravertebral diagnostic block, is surgical section.

Lumbar plexus block

This block is useful in patients suffering from intermittent claudication where reconstructive vascular surgery cannot be carried out because of the generalized vascular disease. In intermittent claudication it is pain which stops the patient walking further and not an insufficient blood supply. If pain can be removed the patient can usually walk a further distance; in other words, their claudication distance can be extended.

The lumbar plexus lies beneath the fascia of the psoas muscle; therefore, solutions injected within the muscle will block the lumbar plexus, and if the concentration of solution is graded so that it will only (or mainly) affect the smaller pain fibres, pain relief without blocking of motor fibres results. The psoas muscle arises from the transverse processes of the lumbar vertebrae, the lateral portions of the intervertebral disc and the lateral borders of the

12th dorsal vertebra and the lumbar vertebrae. The lumbar plexus lies deep and anterior to the transverse processes of the first, second and third lumbar vertebrae in the substance of the psoas major muscle.

An image intensifier is necessary. The needle is inserted as though for a paravertebral block at the L2 level and initially is placed just anterior to the border of the transverse process. A small injection of radio-opaque iophendylate (Myodil) is made and seen on the image intensifier. If the iophendylate spreads into the muscle bundles of the psoas muscle the injection continues, but if it does not then the needle is advanced a little and further injections made until the iophendylate is seen progressing downwards into the muscle.

Various solutions can be used, and 5–7 ml of 7·5 per cent phenol in iophendylate or 10 per cent aqueous solution are advocated by Feldman (1974). The author prefers a larger quantity of more dilute solution and normally uses 10 ml of 1 in 20 phenol in glycerine, using small quantities of iophendylate initially and intermittently to see the progress of the injection. If phenol in glycerine is used, a larger bore needle has to be inserted because of the viscosity of the solution.

Limited regional hip block

This block is advocated by James and Little (1976) for relieving pain in chronic osteoarthritis of the hip. The nerves supplying the structures around the hip joint include the obturator nerve, the femoral nerve, the sciatic nerve, the lumbar sympathetic fibres and the nerve to quadratus femoris. Of these, the obturator nerve and the nerve to quadratus femoris are most important in supplying the sensory nerves to the joint capsule, and a block of these two nerves will, in about 60 per cent of the patients, relieve pain from osteoarthritis. The pain relief is not complete but is of a useful degree. The block can be used also in spastic conditions.

The obturator nerve is blocked in the obturator canal whose upper boundary is the obturator groove on the inferior surface of the superior pubic ramus, the lower boundary being the obturator membrane. A needle is inserted at the mid point between the pubic tubercle and the femoral artery and hits the superior pubic ramus. The needle tip is manœuvred beneath the pubic ramus and advanced upwards almost parallel with the shaft of the femur for about 3 cm. It is then in the obturator foramen.

The nerve to quadratus femoris lies below the piriformis muscle in contact with the deep surface of the sciatic nerve. The patient lies in the prone position with the hip externally rotated; in osteoarthritic patients, this is not always possible. The needle is inserted 5 cm posterior to the greater trochanter of the femur, and a long rigid 15-cm needle is inserted and advanced until it meets the posterior surface of the ischium. It is worked medially, if this is possible, along the bone and this manœuvre places it close to the sciatic nerve and also close to the nerve to quadratus femoris which lies between the bone and the sciatic nerve. An injection of local anaesthetic solution made at this point will diffuse along the surface of the bone and will block the nerve to quadratus femoris. At the same time it will also block the sciatic nerve to a greater or lesser degree and so there will be a transient motor paralysis.

The solutions used for these blocks are simple local anaesthetic agents such as lignocaine or bupivacaine, but the benefits to the patient often last for a few months.

Spinal blocks

There are three varieties of spinal block:
(1) subarachnoid block, (2) epidural block and (3) subdural block.

1. Subarachnoid block

This injection is normally carried out for spinal anaesthesia during operative procedures. In pain treatment work its main value is in the differential spinal blockade which is designed to show if the patient's pain is organic and, if so, through which type of nerve fibres pain is passing. Like all tests designed to decide whether the patient has psychological or organic pain, great care must be taken in interpreting its results. It is of greater value in assessing pain in the lower half of the body than in the upper, for purely technical reasons (Winnie and Collins, 1968).

Subarachnoid spinal puncture is carried out and 5 ml of saline is injected. The patient will appreciate that an injection has been made and is asked after an interval of a few minutes if he has noticed any alteration in his pain. The same procedure is then carried out using 0·2 per cent procaine, 0·5 per cent procaine and 1 per cent procaine. Each of these concentrations will block, respectively, sympathetic nerves, sensory nerves and motor nerves. If the final strength of 1 per cent is not sufficient to block motor nerves in that particular patient, then another injection using 2 per cent procaine can be used. It is not essential to use procaine; any of the modern anaesthetics in equivalent concentrations can be employed. It is fairly obvious that, if the patient has pain relief on the first saline injection or if he obtains no relief after a complete motor block of the spinal cord, then psychological pain is present.

The subarachnoid spinal injection is also of great value for blocking nerves semi-permanently with a neurolytic agent. The commonly used agent is either phenol in glycerine or in iophendylate, but alcohol can also be used and is particularly valuable in certain situations, whilst ammonium chloride is also employed in some clinics.

Phenol

The concentration of phenol in glycerine depends on the level of the spinal cord at which the block is to be made; in sacral and lumbar regions 1 in 20 is used initially, while in the upper dorsal and cervical regions 1 in 15 is safe. This is supposed to be due to the anatomical arrangement of the nerves in relation to the dural cuffs. The lumbar nerves have a long dural cuff, whereas those in the cervical region have a very shallow cuff and thus, the neurolytic agent remains in contact with the lumbar nerve over a longer period of its length than in the cervical region. Phenol in glycerine is a hyperbaric solution and 1 in 20 phenol in glycerine is approximately as strong a neurolytic agent as 1 in 15 in iophendylate in the author's experience. The advantage of phenol in iophendylate is that it can be visualized on x-rays since the iophendylate is radio-opaque; the disadvantage is that it flows much more freely than a glycerine solution.

When this block is carried out, the patient is placed with the painful side dependent and the spinal needle (or needles) inserted at the level of the exit from the bony canal of the nerves to be blocked. The spinal puncture must be clear, free of blood. A small increment of about 0·25 ml of phenol in glycerine is injected after the patient has been tilted posteriorly to 45 degrees. This allows the posterior nerve root to become the most dependent structure in the subarachnoid fluid and the injection of phenol in glycerine will trickle round the dura to this position (Maher, 1955, 1957, 1960). The subarachnoid puncture should be made so that the tip of the needle just enters the dura and any injected material will not drop over the nerve roots of the cauda equina or the cord itself. With the patient conscious, enquiry can be made as to the sensation felt, and the development of analgesia is tested using pinprick sensation. Depending on which way it is desired to extend the effect of the injection, a head-down tilt or headup tilt can be given. It must be remembered that if the neurolytic agent trickles over the S2/S3 nerve roots then bladder complications can result, as the nerve fibres to the bladder pass through these nerve roots.

Alcohol

When used as a neurolytic agent, alcohol tends to produce a neuritis so that pain can result at a later date. Nevertheless, alcohol is a very useful neurolytic agent for subarachnoid blocks, particularly in the mid-dorsal region. The problem in this area of the spinal canal is due to the marked imbrication of the dorsal spines so that it is difficult to place a spinal needle in the subarachnoid space from about T4 to T8. It is by no means impossible but very difficult; if it is attempted, an image intensifier is helpful. When alcohol is to be used, the patient is placed on the non-painful side and tilted anteriorly 45 degrees to bring the posterior nerve root on the painful side uppermost. Alcohol is then injected from above or below this nerve level and, as it is hypobaric, it will flow upwards. When the affected area is placed at the highest point of the subarachnoid space, alcohol floats up to this region. It spreads very rapidly through the cerebrospinal fluid so the position of the patient must be correct before the injection, although small adjustments can be made when successive small increments of alcohol are injected. Sensation to pinprick is checked continuously with the conscious patient.

The patient is kept in position for at least one hour to allow the alcohol to fix and then can be transferred to his bed. The maximal effect of the alcohol is not obtained immediately but develops over 48 hours and occasionally takes up to a week.

Intrathecal phenol drop

This method of producing analgesia in the perineum was devised by Robert Maher (Maher and Mehta, 1977), and is exceedingly valuable for patients who have recurrent carcinoma after an abdominoperineal resection. The principal danger is in allowing the phenol to spread over the nerve roots of the cauda equina if the patient leans forwards while the injection is made. This is avoided by carrying out the lumbar puncture in the normal fashion and then withdrawing the needle until the flow of c.s.f. begins to fall off, showing that the needle is very close to the posterior dura. At this point, with the patient sitting up, he is asked to lean backwards at an angle of about 45 degrees. Less than 0·6 ml of phenol in glycerine, 1 in 20, is injected slowly. If carried out in this fashion the phenol trickles down the posterior dura and will affect only the most dependent of the sacral nerves. If this amount of phenol in glycerine does not produce relief of pain, then on subsequent occasions the quantity can be increased; if this is not sufficient, then the strength can be increased.

2. Epidural block

The epidural space extends between the two layers of the dura mater from the edge of the foramen magnum, where they join, to the sacral hiatus, where they end. An injection made into this space cannot, therefore, extend higher than the foramen magnum. The space contains blood vessels, fat and connective tissue. Laterally, it is continuous with the paravertebral space through the intervertebral foramina.

In the lumbar region the epidural space is triangular in shape, with the apex posteriorly; most epidural blocks are carried out below L3, as the spinal cord does not usually descend below this level. The volume of the space depends on the expansion of the spinal cord, and, thus, there is an increase in size of the epidural space above and below the cervicothoracic enlargement—that is, above C3 and below T4.

There are many techniques of carrying out an epidural injection but they all are dependent upon the fact that there is a reduction of pressure in the epidural space and when a needle enters the epidural space the negative pressure tends to suck in any fluid or air in the needle. Thus, a hanging drop of fluid on the hub of the spinal needle will disappear inwards and an inflated Macintosh balloon fitted to the hub of the needle will deflate. The most common method is to exert manual pressure on the plunger of a syringe filled with saline as the attached epidural needle is inserted at the selected level. As soon as the tip of the needle enters the epidural space, the loss of resistance can be felt and the saline easily injected.

Epidural blocks can be carried out as a 'one shot' method, or a catheter can be inserted through a Tuohy needle and a continuous epidural anaesthetic administered. Great care must be taken that, once the catheter has passed the tip of the needle, it is never withdrawn, because the sharp edge of the Tuohy needle will slice off the end.

This technique of inserting a catheter can be copied to insert temporary stimulating electrodes for diagnostic tests before permanently implanting dorsal column electrodes. Sometimes an incision is made between two vertebral spines down to the interspinous ligament and the electrode then inserted through the Tuohy needle. This is achieved with image intensifier x-ray control and when the electrode is in the correct position, the Tuohy needle can be withdrawn. After a stimulation test confirms the electrode is working and is in the correct position, it is tied down to the ligament with a suture. The wire is then brought out subcutaneously round the side of the body by threading it through an 18-gauge 20 cm needle. The interspinous incision can be closed and the electrode can then be used for a period of at least six weeks. The patient must be warned that, because the electrode tip is free in the epidural space, it may move a little from side to side at times and, therefore, the stimulation sensation may vary a little on occasion.

In chronic pain when all other methods have failed, long-term relief of pain can be obtained by inserting a catheter into the epidural space and administering an intermittent injection of small amounts of local anaesthetic.

3. Subdural injections

This is another of the spinal blocks advocated by Maher and Mehta (1977). Phenol in iophendylate is used for the block so that the injected fluid can be seen on an image intensifier. It is difficult to place the tip of a spinal needle subdurally without entering the subarachnoid space. At this point it lies between the dura and the arachnoid layers. An injection at this level will spread upwards bilaterally between these layers and will also track out long the nerve roots.

There are two methods for inserting the needle for this block. In the first, a spinal needle is inserted into the epidural space and then cautiously advanced until the patient feels a slight sensation of pricking when the needle rests against the dura. A slight rotation of the needle with slight pressure and the point will penetrate the dura without penetrating the arachnoid. An injection of a drop of iophendylate can be seen as a 'spot' in the anteroposterior view on the x-ray screen and further injections will show the radio-opaque material tracking out laterally.

The other method is to perform a subarachnoid block, obtain cerebro-spinal fluid and then withdraw the needle gently until the flow stops. If this is done slowly, the needle tip will remain between the arachnoid and dura in a high proportion of cases and injections will then track between the two layers. The strength of the phenol in iophendylate solution used is 7·5 per cent. It is not difficult to distinguish whether the injection is made in the correct position between the two layers or whether it is epidurally or subarachnoid, as the x-ray appearances are entirely different in the three cases. A lateral x-ray shows the subdural injection as a thin opaque line, extending upwards against gravity. An intrathecal spinal injection will descend with gravity and appear as a series of small beads, while an extradural (epidural) injection appears as an opaque smudge over the whole area of the thecal space.

References

Bridenbaugh, L. D., Moore, D. C. and Campbell, D. D. (1964). Management of upper abdominal cancer pain. *Journal of the American Medical Association* **190**, 877.

Feldman, S. A. (1974) Lumbar sympathetic block. In: *The Treatment of Chronic Pain*, Chapter 6. Ed. by F. D. Hart, M.T.P., Lancaster.

Greenblatt, G. M. and Denson, J. S. (1962). Needle nerve stimulator locator. Nerve blocks with new instrument for locating nerves. *Anaesthesia and Analgesia ... Current Researches* **41**, 599.

James, C. D. T. and Little, T. F. (1976). Regional hip blockade. *Anaesthesia* **31**, 1060–1067.

Maher, R. M. (1955). Relief of pain in incurable cancer. *Lancet* **i**, 836.

Maher, R. M. (1957). Neurone selection in relief of pain; further experiences with intrathecal injections. *Lancet* **i**, 16.

Maher, R. M. (1960). Further experiences with intrathecal and subdural phenol. *Lancet* **i**, 895.

Maher, R. M. and Mehta, M. (1977). Spinal (intrathecal) and extradural analgesia. In *Persistent Pain*, Chapter 4. Ed. by S. Lipton. Academic Press, London and New York.

Sweet, W. H. and Wepsic, J. G. (1974). Controlled thermocoagulation of the trigeminal ganglion and rootlets for differential destruction of pain fibres. *Journal of Neurosurgery* **40**, 143.

Winnie, A. P. and Collins, V. J. (1968). The pain clinic. 1. Differential neurone blockade in pain syndromes of questionable etiology. *Medical Clinics of North America* **52**, 123.

Further reading

Bromage, P. R. (1972). Unblocked segments in epidural analgesia for relief of pain in labour. *British Journal of Anaesthesia* **44**, 676.

Dam, W. and Larsen, J. J. V. (1974). Peripheral nerve blocks in relief of intractable pain. In: *Relief of Intractable Pain*, Chapter 6. Ed. by M. Swerdlow. Excerpta Medica, Amsterdam and London.

Gerbershagen, H. U., Baar, H. A. and Kreuscher, H. (1972). Langzeitnervenblockaden zur Behandlung schwerer Schmerzzustände. 1. Die intrathecale Injektion von Neurolytica. (trans: Long-term nerve blocks in the treatment of severe pain conditions.) *Der Anaesthesist* **21**, 112–121.

Greene, M. N. (1961). Complications of spinal analgesia. *Anesthesiology* **22**, 682.

Eriksson, E. (Ed.). (1969). *Illustrated Handbook in Local Anaesthesia*. I. C. Sørensen & Co. A/S., Copenhagen.

Moore, D. C. (Ed.) (1965). *Regional Block*, 4th edn. Thomas, Springfield, Illinois.

Swerdlow, M. (1974). Intrathecal and extradural block in pain relief. In: *Relief of Intractable Pain*, Chapter 7. Ed. by M. Swerdlow. Excerpta Medica, Amsterdam and London.

Index